The Basic Breathwork Book

The Basic Breathwork Book

Ravenwood Press

CONTENTS

Introduction to Breathwork

Chapter 1: Introduction to Breathwork
Understanding Breathwork

Breathwork, at its core, is the practice of conscious control of your breath. It's about harnessing the power of the most basic and essential function of life - breathing - and using it as a tool to enhance physical, emotional, and spiritual well-being.

While breathwork has seen a surge in popularity in recent years, it isn't a new concept. The idea of using breath control to improve health and consciousness can be traced back thousands of years and is a common thread in many ancient philosophies and healing practices.

Historical Background and Origins of Breathwork

The roots of breathwork are as deep as they are widespread, spanning across time and cultures. The yogis of ancient India, for example, developed a practice called Pranayama, a Sanskrit term where 'prana' means life force and 'yama' means control.

By consciously altering their breathing patterns, these ancient practitioners believed they could control their life force, improving health and promoting spiritual growth.

Similarly, the Tibetan practice of Tummo involves controlling the breath to generate body heat, aiding meditation and spiritual development. These are just two examples among many, demonstrating how intrinsic the link between breath and well-being is across different cultures and philosophies.

Different Forms of Breathwork

Today, numerous forms of breathwork exist, each with its own unique focus and method. Pranayama, with its origins in ancient yogic traditions, remains popular. In addition, there's Holotropic Breathwork, a practice developed by psychiatrist Stanislav Grof designed to achieve self-understanding and spiritual growth through non-ordinary states of consciousness. The Wim Hof Method, named after its Dutch creator, uses breathwork techniques to influence the body's immune response and resilience. Rebirthing Breathwork focuses on releasing stored emotional trauma to facilitate psychological and spiritual growth.

While these practices differ in their methods and goals, they all share a common principle: the conscious control of breath can bring about significant benefits for mind, body, and spirit.

Potential Benefits of Breathwork

The potential benefits of breathwork are vast and varied, ranging from physical enhancements such as improved cardiovascular function and immune response, to mental benefits such as stress reduction, improved focus, and increased emotional stability.

Studies have shown that breathwork can help regulate the body's autonomic nervous system, which controls key functions like heart rate, digestion, and the stress response. By learning to control our breathing, we can potentially influence these automatic functions, promoting a healthier physiological state and improved mental well-being.

On a deeper level, many practitioners use breathwork as a tool for spiritual exploration, facilitating a deeper connection with the self and the universe.

Personal Journey with Breathwork

My journey with breathwork began when I was searching for natural ways to manage stress and improve focus. As I delved into the practice, I experienced first-hand the transformative power of breathwork. It helped me manage my stress levels, improved my mental clarity, and even brought about profound spiritual experiences. This personal transformation was what inspired me to share the power of breathwork with others through this book.

In the chapters to come, we'll delve into the science behind breathwork, learn different breathing techniques, and explore how you can incorporate breathwork into your daily routine to improve your physical, emotional, and spiritual well-being.

2

The Science Behind Breathwork

Chapter 2: The Science Behind Breathwork
The Physiology of Breathing
The Basic Process of Breathing

The ability to breathe is a miraculous and complex process. The simple act of inhaling and exhaling supports life, facilitating the critical exchange of gases needed for our survival. This section examines the process of breathing, breaking down its two main steps—inhaling and exhaling—and delving into the essential role each plays in sustaining life.

Inhalation: Drawing Oxygen into Our Lungs

Inhalation is the first half of the breathing cycle. It begins when we contract our diaphragm, a dome-shaped muscle situated below the lungs. As the diaphragm contracts and moves downward, it increases the space within our chest cavity. This expansion results in a drop in internal air pressure compared to the external environment, and to equalize the pressure, air rushes into our lungs.

This air is rich in oxygen, a gas crucial for our survival. Once in the lungs, this oxygen-laden air travels down progressively smaller tubes—starting from the bronchi, then into the bronchioles—until it reaches the alveoli.

The alveoli are tiny, balloon-like structures where the critical gas exchange occurs. Oxygen in the air we've inhaled diffuses through the thin walls of the alveoli and into the surrounding capillaries. Here, it enters the bloodstream to be transported to every cell in the body.

Exhalation: Removing Carbon Dioxide from Our Bodies

Exhalation, the second half of the breathing cycle, is essentially the reverse process of inhalation. It begins when the diaphragm relaxes and moves upward, decreasing the space within the chest cavity. This decrease in volume leads to an increase in internal air pressure compared to the external environment. To equalize this pressure difference, air is pushed out from the lungs and back into the environment.

This exhaled air carries with it carbon dioxide, a waste product of the body's metabolic processes. Like oxygen, carbon dioxide also diffuses from the bloodstream into the alveoli, but in the opposite direction—moving from the blood in the capillaries, through the alveolar walls, and into the air within the alveoli. From here, it's expelled from the body when we exhale.

Conclusion

The process of breathing—inhaling and exhaling—is a

beautiful orchestration of muscle movement and gas exchange that keeps us alive. Understanding this continuous cycle illuminates not just how we breathe, but why we breathe, providing us with a foundational understanding of one of our body's most vital processes.

Respiratory Anatomy

The journey of air as we inhale and exhale is facilitated by an intricate network of structures constituting our respiratory system. Each component, from our nasal cavity to the smallest alveolus in our lungs, plays a vital role in sustaining life. This section aims to delve into these structures and shed light on their unique functions within the broader respiratory system.

The Nasal Cavity and the Mouth

Air's journey begins at the nasal cavity or the mouth, serving as primary entry and exit points. Beyond being mere gateways, the nasal cavity adds additional functions—it warms, humidifies, and filters the incoming air, preparing it for a safe journey down the respiratory tract.

The Trachea and Bronchi

From the nasal cavity or mouth, air descends into the trachea. Akin to a tree trunk, the trachea branches into two bronchi, each leading to a lung. The bronchi then split into smaller bronchioles, forming a tree-like network that escorts air deep into the lungs.

The Lungs and Alveoli

The lungs are the epicenters of respiration. Each lung houses millions of alveoli, which are tiny, balloon-like structures where the crucial gas exchange occurs. Each alveolus is wrapped by a dense network of capillaries, placing the incoming air in close proximity to the bloodstream. This strategic arrangement facilitates the efficient diffusion of oxygen into the blood and the expulsion of carbon dioxide from it.

The Diaphragm

Residing beneath the lungs is the diaphragm—a robust, dome-shaped muscle that plays a pivotal role in breathing. The diaphragm's rhythmic contractions and relaxations drive the ebb and flow of air in and out of the lungs by creating necessary pressure changes within the chest cavity.

Conclusion

From the warming of air in the nasal cavity to the critical exchange of gases in the alveoli, each component of the respiratory system works cohesively, contributing to the overall process of respiration. Recognizing these structures and understanding their functions paints a vivid picture of our body's incredible capacity to sustain life. This knowledge not only evokes awe at our body's complexity and efficiency but also underscores the importance of maintaining respiratory health.

Chemistry of Breathing

Breathing's simplicity belies a complex biochemical process that underpins life. More than mere gas displacement, it involves a delicate interplay of oxygen and carbon dioxide within our bloodstream. In this section, we will delve into this intricate process, outlining how oxygen fuels cellular metabolism and how carbon dioxide—a byproduct of this process— is expelled from our bodies.

Oxygen's Journey: From Inhalation to Cellular Metabolism

The air we inhale contains about 21% oxygen. As we breathe in, oxygen travels through the respiratory tract, ultimately reaching the alveoli in the lungs. Here, oxygen diffuses across the alveolar wall into the surrounding capillaries. Once in the bloodstream, oxygen binds with hemoglobin, a protein in red blood cells, forming oxyhemoglobin. These oxygen-laden red blood cells are then transported throughout the body, delivering oxygen to every cell.

Carbon Dioxide's Journey: From Cells to Exhalation

Cellular metabolism, particularly the process known as cellular respiration, generates energy by breaking down glucose in the presence of oxygen, producing carbon dioxide as a waste product. This carbon dioxide diffuses into the bloodstream, where it's primarily carried in the form of bicarbonate ions. The blood, rich in carbon dioxide, returns to the lungs, where the carbon dioxide diffuses back into the alveoli to be exhaled, completing the gas exchange cycle.

Regulation of Breathing

Breathing's rate and depth are mostly automatic, regulated by the respiratory center in the brainstem. But this autonomic process is far from rigid—it dynamically adjusts to environmental demands and internal changes to maintain the body's homeostasis. In this section, we will explore how our bodies regulate breathing and respond to various influencing factors.

The Role of the Respiratory Center

The respiratory center, located in the medulla oblongata of the brainstem, plays a pivotal role in regulating breath. It continually receives information about the body's levels of oxygen, carbon dioxide, and blood pH, mainly from chemoreceptors in the carotid arteries and the aorta. Elevated carbon dioxide levels or a decrease in blood pH triggers the respiratory center to increase the breathing rate and depth to expel carbon dioxide and restore balance.

Influencing Factors on Breathing

Beyond the primary drive to balance blood gases and pH, breathing can also be influenced by a variety of factors. Physical activity, for example, accelerates metabolic activity, producing more carbon dioxide and requiring increased oxygen intake, thus increasing the breathing rate. Emotional states, like stress or anxiety, can also alter our breathing patterns. Finally, health conditions such as respiratory diseases, heart conditions, and certain medications can affect the rate and depth of breathing.

Breathing is thus a responsive and adaptive process, finely tuned to meet our body's needs and respond to our environment, demonstrating its critical role in maintaining life and health.

The Connection Between Breath and the Nervous System

Understanding the Autonomic Nervous System

The autonomic nervous system (ANS) is an intricate part of our nervous system operating largely beneath our conscious awareness. It regulates vital functions, from our heart rate to our digestion, ensuring our internal systems function smoothly. In this section, we will explore the ANS, particularly its two main branches—the sympathetic and parasympathetic nervous systems—and how they contribute to our physiological responses and overall well-being.

The Sympathetic and Parasympathetic Nervous Systems

The ANS consists of two primary branches: the sympathetic nervous system (SNS) and the parasympathetic nervous system (PNS). The SNS is often referred to as the 'fight or flight' system. It primes the body for action, increasing heart rate, dilating pupils, and mobilizing energy reserves, among other things. The PNS, on the other hand, is associated with 'rest and digest' or 'feed and breed' responses. It promotes relaxation, digestion, and energy conservation. Both systems operate in a complementary manner to maintain the body's internal equilibrium, or homeostasis.

Breath and the Sympathetic Nervous System

Breathing, though a seemingly simple process, is intimately tied to our sympathetic nervous system. Changes in our breathing patterns often reflect shifts in our internal physiological state, particularly during moments of stress or danger. In this section, we'll delve into the SNS's impact on our breathing and its broader implications for our health and well-being.

The 'Fight or Flight' Response and Breathing

When the SNS is activated—often due to perceived threats or stress—it triggers a cascade of physiological changes to prepare the body for potential 'fight or flight.' One significant change is in our breathing patterns. The rate and depth of our breaths increase to supply the body with more oxygen and expel carbon dioxide faster, fueling potential physical exertion.

Breathing as a Reflection of our Physiological State

Our breath, thus, acts as a mirror to our internal state. Rapid, shallow breathing often indicates a state of stress or anxiety, reflecting an activated SNS. Understanding this connection between breath and the nervous system can inform various approaches to managing stress and promoting relaxation, underscoring breath's critical role in our overall well-being.

Breath and the Parasympathetic Nervous System

The parasympathetic nervous system (PNS), often described as the 'rest and digest' system, plays a crucial role in promoting relaxation and recovery in our bodies. It facilitates slower, deeper breathing and a range of other physiological processes geared towards restoring and conserving energy. In this section, we'll delve into the intricate relationship between our breath and the PNS and how this connection contributes to our overall well-being.

The 'Rest and Digest' Response and Breathing

Upon activation, the PNS initiates a series of physiological changes designed to promote relaxation and recovery. These changes include slowing the heart rate, stimulating digestion, and enabling slower, deeper breathing. This shift in breathing allows for more efficient gas exchange and can induce a sense of calm and tranquility, making it a powerful tool for stress management and relaxation.

Conscious Breathing and Autonomic Regulation

While the autonomic nervous system operates largely below the threshold of conscious perception, we do have control over one of its functions: our breath. Through conscious modulation of our breath, we can influence our physiological state, either stimulating the parasympathetic response to promote relaxation or invoking the sympathetic response to boost alertness. This section will provide a comprehensive understanding of this autonomic regulation process, highlighting the role of breathwork as a tool for managing our physiological and psychological states.

Breathwork and Autonomic Regulation

Consciously altering our breath can influence our autonomic nervous system, allowing us to tap into its regulatory power. For instance, slow, deep, diaphragmatic breathing tends to stimulate the PNS, promoting relaxation and reducing stress. On the other hand, faster, shallower breathing can activate the SNS, enhancing alertness and energy. Understanding and applying these principles can transform breathwork from a simple exercise into a powerful tool for health and well-being.

Practical Applications

Harnessing the power of breath for autonomic regulation requires consistent practice and mindful awareness. With patience and persistence, conscious breathing can become a part of our daily routines, providing us with a readily accessible means of managing stress, promoting relaxation, and enhancing our overall quality of life. As we delve further into the world of breathwork, we'll explore various techniques and practices to help integrate this powerful tool into your daily life.

Breathwork for Stress and Relaxation

Breathwork can be a powerful tool in managing stress and promoting relaxation. Specific breathing techniques, such as diaphragmatic and box breathing, can effectively stimulate the parasympathetic nervous system, inducing a state of calm and relaxation. In this section, we'll explore the science behind these techniques, discussing their physiological impacts and offering practical guidance for effective use.

Diaphragmatic and Box Breathing

Diaphragmatic breathing involves deep, slow breaths that expand the diaphragm, promoting a slower heart rate and lower blood pressure. Similarly, box breathing—a technique that involves equal periods of inhaling, holding the breath, exhaling, and holding the breath again—can help in activating the parasympathetic response. These techniques not only reduce physical symptoms of stress but also foster a calm and relaxed mental state.

Practical Applications

Learning and applying these techniques requires practice, but over time, they can become a readily accessible tool for managing stress and promoting relaxation. Through step-by-step guidance, we'll explain how to incorporate these techniques into your daily routine effectively.

Breathwork for Energy and Focus

While many breathwork techniques aim to induce relaxation, others are designed to stimulate energy and focus. These methods often involve quicker, more forceful breaths and can activate the sympathetic nervous system, thereby enhancing physical readiness and mental acuity. This section will delve into these energizing techniques, the physiological processes they trigger, and provide practical tips for their implementation.

Energizing Breathwork Techniques

Certain breathwork techniques, such as the Wim Hof Method or Bhastrika pranayama (a yogic breath of fire), involve quick, forceful breaths that can stimulate the sympathetic nervous system. This stimulation leads to a host of physiological changes, including increased heart rate and enhanced alertness, effectively boosting energy levels and focus.

Practical Applications

Understanding and correctly applying these techniques can be an effective strategy for enhancing energy and focus when needed. Whether it's preparing for a workout, an important meeting, or a creative endeavor, these techniques can provide a natural and accessible boost to your physical readiness and mental acuity. Through guided instructions, we'll show you how to safely and effectively incorporate these energizing techniques into your lifestyle.

Integrating Breathwork into Daily Life

With an understanding of how breathwork influences the mind and body, we can apply this powerful tool across various aspects of daily life. Breathwork can be used to start the day on a calm note, provide an energy boost when needed, or assist in transitioning to a relaxed state before sleep. In this section, we'll outline practical strategies for incorporating breathwork into your daily routine, enhancing your well being.

Starting the Day with Calming Breathwork

Beginning the day with a calming breathwork routine can set a peaceful tone for the hours to come. Techniques such as diaphragmatic or box breathing can help to center the mind, ground the body, and prepare you for the day ahead.

Using Breathwork for an Energy Boost

Rather than reaching for a caffeinated drink when afternoon fatigue hits, consider using invigorating breathwork techniques. Practices such as the Wim Hof Method or Bhastrika pranayama can stimulate the sympathetic nervous system, enhancing energy and focus.

Preparing for Sleep with Relaxing Breathwork

Deep, slow breathwork patterns can be an excellent tool for preparing the body for sleep. These techniques, like the 4-7-8 breathing practice, can stimulate the parasympathetic nervous system, reducing heart rate, promoting relaxation, and preparing the body for a restful night's sleep.

Conclusion

Breathwork, with its multifaceted influence on the mind and body, can be a valuable addition to daily life. By learning to harness the power of the breath, we can foster a sense of inner balance, enhancing overall well being and making each day more meaningful.

Scientific Studies and Evidence on the Benefits of Breathwork

Breathwork for Stress and Anxiety

Research has repeatedly shown the benefits of breathwork for mitigating stress and anxiety. Studies using various breathwork techniques have reported reductions in symptoms of anxiety and improved responses to stress. Participants have noted lower levels of perceived stress and enhanced feelings of calm and relaxation. This research highlights the potential for breathwork as a self-regulated tool for managing stress and anxiety, offering an accessible, cost-effective complement to traditional therapeutic approaches.

Breathwork for Cardiovascular Health

Breathwork also holds promise for cardiovascular health. Research has indicated that certain breathwork techniques can help lower blood pressure, enhance heart rate variability, and potentially decrease the risk of cardiovascular disease. These studies underscore the potential role of breathwork in maintaining cardiovascular health and preventing disease, opening up new avenues for holistic and integrative health strategies.

Breathwork for Cognitive Performance

The potential benefits of breathwork extend to cognitive performance as well. Research has suggested that certain breathwork practices can improve focus, memory, and other cognitive functions. By bolstering attention and enhancing mindfulness, these techniques can lead to improvements in various cognitive domains, pointing to the potential of breathwork as a tool for cognitive enhancement and overall mental well-being.

Breathwork and the Immune Response

Emerging research suggests that breathwork could play a role in boosting the immune response. Some studies have shown that certain breathing techniques can influence the immune system, potentially reducing inflammation and promoting the release of immune cells. While the mechanisms are not entirely understood, it is speculated that the relaxation response induced by breathwork might suppress stress-induced inflammation and enhance immune function. These promising findings indicate that breathwork may not only improve mental and cardiovascular health, but could also have significant implications for overall immune health and disease resistance.

The Psychological Aspects of Breathwork
Breathwork for Emotional Awareness

Breathwork can serve as a powerful tool for enhancing emotional awareness. By focusing on the rhythm and sensations of our breath, we can cultivate a stronger connection with our inner emotional landscapes. This awareness can help us more clearly identify and understand our emotions, ultimately assisting us in better managing them. Moreover, increased emotional awareness can foster improved emotional intelligence, nurturing healthier relationships with ourselves and with others. In this section, we will explore the connection between breathwork and emotional awareness, illuminating the scientific understanding of this relationship and providing practical strategies for employing breathwork in the pursuit of greater emotional insight.

Breathwork for Stress Management

Breathwork is a potent tool for stress management. Beyond initiating physiological relaxation responses, it also influences our psychological responses to stress, helping us foster resilience and a balanced perspective. Specific breathwork practices can help shift our perspective from reactive to responsive, allowing us to navigate stressful situations with greater ease and poise. In this section, we delve into the psychological benefits of breathwork in stress management. We'll discuss relevant theories and research that substantiate these benefits and provide practical strategies for integrating these techniques into stress-inducing scenarios.

Breathwork for Self-Discovery and Personal Growth

Breathwork transcends mere physiological and emotional benefits, becoming a vehicle for self-discovery and personal growth. Certain breathwork practices have the potential to catalyze transformative experiences. These experiences can offer profound insights into our patterns of thought, deeply ingrained beliefs, and habitual behaviors. In turn, such self-awareness can serve as a springboard for personal evolution and growth. In this section, we'll delve into this profound dimension of breathwork, exploring the ways various techniques can foster self-understanding and personal growth. We will also offer guidance on how to safely and effectively embark on this transformative journey.

Basic Breathing Techniques

Chapter 3: Basic Breathing Techniques
An Overview of Basic Breathwork Techniques
The Importance of Basic Techniques

Breathwork, like any other discipline, requires a solid foundation to effectively progress. Fundamental breathwork techniques are essential in this regard, serving to familiarize us with conscious breathing and teaching us to control the depth, rhythm, and pace of our breaths. In this section, we'll discuss why mastering these foundational techniques is critical, exploring the key skills they cultivate and how they lay the groundwork for more advanced breathwork practices.

Types of Basic Breathwork Techniques

There are numerous basic breathwork techniques, each offering distinct benefits and experiences. Some of these include diaphragmatic breathing, box breathing, and the 4-7-8 breathing technique, among others. This section will introduce these techniques, discussing their specific processes and unique attributes.

The Role of Attention in Basic Breathwork Techniques

Attention plays a vital role in basic breathwork techniques. By intentionally directing our focus to our breath, we do more than just physically alter our breathing pattern; we also train our minds to be more present and focused. In this section, we'll delve into the concept of attention within breathwork, discussing how it amplifies the effectiveness of the practice and contributes to its psychological benefits.

From Basic to Advanced: The Breathwork Journey

While basic techniques are a starting point, they are also the stepping stones to more advanced practices. As we get comfortable with these basic techniques, we can start to explore more complex forms of breathwork that offer different experiences and benefits. In this concluding section, we will discuss how to progress from basic to advanced techniques, offering guidance on when and how to make this transition.

Box Breathing

Box breathing, also known as square breathing, is a widely practiced breathwork technique that is both simple and effective. Originally stemming from Pranayama yoga, it has since been adopted by a diverse range of professionals, from athletes to military personnel, due to its ability to enhance focus, alleviate stress, and improve performance. In this section, we'll unpack the concept of box breathing, delve into its processes, and discuss the principles underlying its effectiveness.

The Process of Box Breathing

The terms "box" or "square" in box breathing are derived

from the equal time allotment given to each of its four phases —inhalation, hold, exhalation, and hold. In this part of the guide, we'll provide a detailed, step-by-step walk-through of box breathing, starting with the initial preparations and moving on to the actual breathing process. We'll cover practical aspects like finding a comfortable posture, setting a suitable pace for your breaths, and visualizing the "box" to help time your breaths accurately.

Benefits of Box Breathing

Box breathing boasts an array of benefits, ranging from stress reduction and improved focus, to an enhanced mind-body connection and better sleep quality. In this section, we'll delve deep into these benefits, referring to scientific studies where applicable to substantiate these claims. The goal of this section is to equip readers with a comprehensive understanding of how and why box breathing can positively influence their well being.

Applying Box Breathing in Everyday Life

The simplicity of box breathing belies its versatility as a tool that can be effectively utilized in a myriad of situations. Whether serving as a stress-reliever during high-pressure moments, an aid to concentration during tasks that demand focus, or a calming pre-sleep routine promoting better rest, box breathing has the potential to significantly improve daily life. In this section, we will discuss how to seamlessly incorporate box breathing into various aspects of your everyday routine and provide tips to maximize its benefits.

Diaphragmatic Breathing

Diaphragmatic breathing, commonly known as belly

breathing, is a natural and efficient way of breathing that involves the diaphragm—a large muscle located between the chest and the abdomen. This technique encourages full oxygen exchange, slows the heartbeat, and can help stabilize blood pressure. In this section, we'll explore the basics of diaphragmatic breathing, including its roots in ancient practices, and its modern-day relevance and applications.

The Process of Diaphragmatic Breathing

Although diaphragmatic breathing comes naturally to us as infants, many adults unlearn this habit and tend to take shallow, chest-based breaths—especially under stress. The practice of diaphragmatic breathing involves relearning to breathe deeply into the belly. In this part, we will guide you through the process of diaphragmatic breathing, explaining how to locate and engage the diaphragm, establish correct breathing patterns, and ways to practice this technique effectively.

Benefits of Diaphragmatic Breathing

Diaphragmatic breathing brings a plethora of health benefits, including increased relaxation, reduced stress, improved lung function, and enhanced core muscle stability. In this section, we will delve into these benefits in detail, providing insights into the scientific and physiological aspects that underpin these outcomes. We will also explore the therapeutic applications of diaphragmatic breathing in managing various health conditions, such as chronic obstructive pulmonary disease (COPD) and anxiety disorders.

Applying Diaphragmatic Breathing in Daily Life

The versatility of diaphragmatic breathing makes it an invaluable tool that can be incorporated into our everyday routines. Whether utilized during moments of stress, integrated into a daily relaxation practice, or employed to enhance physical activities like singing or sports, diaphragmatic breathing is a skill with a wide array of applications. In this section, we will offer guidance on recognizing opportunities for practicing and benefiting from diaphragmatic breathing in everyday life, and provide practical suggestions for incorporating this technique into various scenarios.

4-7-8 Breathing

The 4-7-8 breathing technique, often referred to as the "relaxing breath," is a method that was brought into the mainstream by Dr. Andrew Weil. With its origins in the ancient yogic technique known as pranayama, 4-7-8 breathing is recognized for its potential to induce a calming and tranquilizing effect on the nervous system. In this segment, we will delve into the foundations and principles of 4-7-8 breathing, elucidating the significance of the numbers and their integral role in the practice.

The Process of 4-7-8 Breathing

4-7-8 breathing is a relatively simple technique that involves inhaling for a count of 4, holding the breath for a count of 7, and then exhaling for a count of 8. In this section, we will furnish a thorough, step-by-step guide to practicing 4-7-8 breathing. We will provide advice on counting the breaths, adapting the practice for comfort, and ensuring the proper breathing form is adhered to—specifically, diaphragmatic breathing.

Benefits of 4-7-8 Breathing

The 4-7-8 breathing technique has been praised for its capacity to alleviate stress, enhance sleep quality, manage cravings, and control or diminish anger responses. In this part, we will scrutinize each of these benefits, referencing both scientific research and anecdotal evidence to offer a well-rounded perspective of the advantages this technique can provide.

Applying 4-7-8 Breathing in Everyday Life

In the concluding section, we will address the incorporation of 4-7-8 breathing into everyday life. This technique can be employed anywhere, at any time, making it a powerful tool for immediate stress relief. From countering sleeplessness to diffusing tension during a challenging conversation, we will furnish practical examples and tips to maximize the effectiveness of 4-7-8 breathing in day-to-day scenarios.

The Benefits and Best Use Cases for Each Technique

Breathwork, despite its shared focus on controlled, mindful breathing, encompasses a wide array of techniques that offer diverse benefits and applications. These techniques vary in their effects based on factors such as rhythm, depth of breath, point of focus, and complexity of the practice. In this section, we'll provide a summary of the unique benefits and best use cases for each of the breathwork techniques we've discussed in this guide: Box Breathing, Diaphragmatic Breathing, and the 4-7-8 Breathing method.

Box Breathing

Box Breathing is a versatile technique with potential to manage stress, improve focus, and increase overall mindfulness. Its balanced, rhythmic pattern is particularly useful in situations requiring calm and concentration. Whether you're preparing for a challenging presentation, winding down before bed, or looking for a mid-day mental refresh amidst a busy workday, Box Breathing can be a go-to resource.

Diaphragmatic Breathing

Diaphragmatic Breathing, or 'belly breathing', is primarily aimed at fostering deep relaxation and improving physical health. This technique, characterized by deep, full breaths, is an excellent method for stress management, sleep improvement, and enhancing lung function, particularly beneficial for individuals with respiratory conditions. It can be seamlessly integrated into a daily relaxation routine, or used to augment the benefits of other activities like yoga, meditation, or even singing.

4-7-8 Breathing

The 4-7-8 Breathing Technique is a powerful tool for rapid stress relief and facilitating better sleep. It is especially useful in situations where immediate relaxation is necessary - be it anxiety-induced moments, difficulties in falling asleep, or dealing with intense cravings. Given its simplicity, the 4-7-8 technique is a ready-at-hand solution for on-the-spot stress relief, whether you're in a tense meeting, stuck in traffic, or navigating a difficult conversation.

Tips for Beginners

Understanding the Importance of Breathwork

Before immersing in breathwork, one must understand its profound significance. Your breath is not just a life-sustaining process; it's a potent tool that can be harnessed for health improvement, stress reduction, and heightened self-awareness. We'll recap the many benefits of breathwork, backed by scientific evidence, to emphasize its potential impact on physical and mental well-being.

Creating a Comfortable Environment

A quiet, comfortable environment significantly enhances the breathwork experience. This space can be a tranquil corner of your room, a cozy spot by a window, or any place where you feel at ease and undisturbed. We'll suggest some ways to create a conducive breathwork space, incorporating elements like cushions, blankets, and calming aids such as candles or soft music.

Starting Slow and Steady

Breathwork is a journey, not a race. Initiating with a slow and steady approach prevents feelings of overwhelm and allows for the establishment of a strong foundation. We'll guide you on how to start with short, manageable sessions, gradually escalating the duration and complexity as your comfort level and proficiency increase.

Practicing Regularly

Consistency is the linchpin of successful breathwork. Like physical exercise, the benefits of breathwork compound over time with consistent practice. We'll offer strategies to maintain a regular breathwork routine, such as incorporating breathwork into existing daily routines or using reminders and apps to stay on track.

Overcoming Common Challenges

Finally, we'll tackle common challenges beginners may encounter, like discomfort, dizziness, or difficulty in concentrating, and provide solutions to surmount them. It's important to remember that these experiences are normal and usually wane with practice. We'll also suggest possible modifications or alternatives if certain techniques prove uncomfortable.

4

Advanced Breathing Techniques

Chapter 4: Advanced Breathing Techniques
An Overview of Advanced Breathwork Techniques

As we delve deeper into the realm of breathwork, we encounter advanced techniques that, while requiring more mastery and control, offer the potential for profound experiences and deep self-exploration. Building on the foundational skills we have established, this section explores advanced breathwork techniques, distinguishing their unique characteristics and showcasing how they elevate our breathwork practice.

Characteristics of Advanced Breathwork Techniques

Advanced breathwork techniques often involve intricate breathing patterns, longer durations, and may integrate elements such as breath retention, forceful exhales, or rapid inhales. Certain techniques are designed to induce altered states of consciousness or facilitate emotional catharsis. While these practices can be transformative, they demand a higher degree of awareness and familiarity with breath control.

Building Upon Foundational Skills

The basic techniques we've discussed form the foundation upon which advanced breathwork is built. Skills such as focused attention on the breath, controlled inhalation and exhalation, and understanding the impacts of different breathing patterns on the body and mind are all critical in practicing advanced techniques. These intricate methods often amplify the effects experienced with basic techniques, fostering deeper relaxation, heightened focus, and profound spiritual experiences.

Safety and Guidance in Advanced Breathwork

Advanced breathwork, while holding immense potential for personal growth and discovery, should be approached with an understanding of safety. Some techniques can be intense, necessitating the guidance of a knowledgeable instructor, especially for beginners. We'll delve deeper into safety considerations in this chapter.

As we navigate this chapter, we'll study several advanced techniques, including Holotropic Breathwork, the Wim Hof Method, and Sudarshan Kriya. We'll explore their origins, practices, benefits, and safety considerations. With time, practice, and patience, these advanced techniques can serve as powerful tools for personal transformation and well-being.

Pranayama Techniques

Pranayama, a term derived from Sanskrit, translates to "life force extension" and plays a pivotal role in the yogic practices of ancient India. This art of breath control goes beyond simple inhalation and exhalation, aiming to expand the prana, or life force, within an individual. In this section, we'll familiarize ourselves with several fundamental Pranayama techniques, exploring their methods, implications, and the unique benefits they offer.

Nadi Shodhana (Alternate Nostril Breathing)

Nadi Shodhana, also known as Alternate Nostril Breathing, is a Pranayama technique revered for its calming and balancing effects. The term 'Nadi' translates to 'channel' or 'flow,' and 'Shodhana' means 'purification.' Therefore, the practice of Nadi Shodhana centers around purifying and harmonizing the energy channels within the body. This technique involves a precise pattern of inhaling and exhaling through the nostrils. We'll provide detailed instructions to guide you through Nadi Shodhana, highlighting its potential to foster stress relief, deep relaxation, and mental clarity.

Kapalabhati (Skull Shining Breath)

Kapalabhati, known in English as Skull Shining Breath, is a dynamic and invigorating Pranayama technique. The term 'Kapala' translates to 'skull,' while 'bhati' signifies 'shining,' reflecting the technique's energizing and illuminating nature. The practice of Kapalabhati involves a sequence of forceful exhalations followed by passive inhalations. We'll delve into the methodology of Kapalabhati, discussing its benefits related to purifying the lungs, energizing the body, and enhancing focus.

Bhastrika (Bellows Breath)

Bhastrika, commonly referred to as Bellows Breath, is another profound Pranayama technique. The term 'Bhastrika' translates to 'bellows,' reflecting the technique's warming and invigorating properties, much like a bellows used to stoke fire. This method involves rhythmic inhalations and exhalations that can generate heat and elevate energy within the body. In the following sections, we'll guide you through the practice of Bhastrika, elucidating its benefits, which include improved circulation, heightened alertness, and a potential increase in metabolic function.

Bhramari (Bee Breathing)

Bhramari Pranayama, often known as Bee Breathing, derives its name from the distinctive humming sound made during the practice, reminiscent of a buzzing bee. Bhramari is a grounding technique celebrated for its calming influence and ability to mitigate stress and anxiety. We'll walk you through the step-by-step practice of Bhramari, emphasizing its potential to foster tranquility and enhance mental clarity.

The Holistic Impact of Pranayama

Pranayama is more than a set of breathing exercises; it's a comprehensive approach to holistic well-being. Although each pranayama technique possesses distinct benefits, collectively, they promote a holistic sense of physical and mental equilibrium. Incorporating pranayama into your daily routine can help manage stress, improve focus, and guide you towards a balanced, enriched state of existence. As we delve deeper into advanced breathwork techniques, we'll uncover more transformative practices, propelling your breathwork journey to uncharted territories.

Holotropic Breathwork

Holotropic Breathwork is a unique, transformative, and

therapeutically potent breathwork technique. It was conceived in the mid-20th century by psychiatrist Dr. Stanislav Grof and is designed to catalyze self-discovery, healing, and spiritual insight by combining specific breathing patterns, music, and bodywork. Unlike other breathwork techniques we've encountered, Holotropic Breathwork aims to induce non-ordinary states of consciousness, signifying its deep potency and transformative ability.

Understanding Holotropic Breathwork

Administered in group sessions under the supervision of trained professionals, Holotropic Breathwork encompasses three key elements: accelerated breathing, evocative music, and concentrated bodywork. The foundational belief is that our psyche inherently possesses the capacity for guidance towards healing and wholeness, which this intense process allows us to access. We'll delve into each element, explaining how they contribute to the holistic experience of Holotropic Breathwork.

Potential Benefits and Applications

Holotropic Breathwork serves as a tool for self-exploration, therapy, and spiritual growth. Participants often report profound emotional release, heightened self-awareness, and transformative insights during and after sessions. Some individuals even experience vivid imagery, recollections, and symbolic phenomena, offering fresh perspectives on their life. We'll elaborate on these potential benefits and applications, presenting anecdotal accounts and scientific evidence supporting this practice.

Safety and Precautions

Despite its potential advantages, Holotropic Breathwork is a rigorous practice and isn't suitable for everyone. People with specific medical conditions—including cardiovascular disease, severe hypertension, and certain psychiatric disorders—should refrain from this practice. Furthermore, even for those in good health, it's crucial to perform Holotropic Breathwork under the supervision of a trained professional. We'll address the necessary precautions, the significance of a secure and supportive environment, and what to anticipate during a session.

Conclusion Holotropic Breathwork stands apart as a unique and profound technique within the breathwork realm. Its ability to facilitate deep psychological and spiritual experiences sets it apart from many other practices. However, this technique demands care, preparation, and professional facilitation. With appropriate guidance and respect for the process, Holotropic Breathwork can offer a deeply transformative journey into the self. As we advance, we'll uncover other advanced breathwork techniques that can further deepen your understanding and mastery of this powerful practice.

Wim Hof Method

The Wim Hof Method, named after its Dutch creator, a renowned extreme athlete dubbed 'The Iceman,' has attracted significant interest in recent years. This unique method fuses controlled breathing, exposure to cold, and meditation. Wim Hof's extraordinary feats, including climbing Mount Everest wearing only shorts and running a marathon in the scorching Namibian desert without water, have ignited global curiosity. Hof attributes his seemingly superhuman achievements to his eponymous method, which he believes allows him to modulate his body's responses to extreme conditions.

Understanding the Wim Hof Method

The Wim Hof Method incorporates three fundamental elements. The first component is a distinctive breathing technique, somewhat akin to Pranayama and Tummo (inner heat) Meditation, yet singular in its approach and objectives. The second aspect involves gradual, controlled exposure to cold conditions, such as icy showers or ice baths. The final element is meditation, which focuses the mind and enriches the overall experience. We will delve into each of these components, explaining their roles and how to safely implement them.

Potential Benefits and Applications

Advocates of the Wim Hof Method report a broad spectrum of benefits, encompassing enhanced energy, an improved immune response, better sleep, and alleviated symptoms of specific ailments. Numerous scientific studies have scrutinized the method, some of which have provided evidence substantiating these claims. We will dissect these potential benefits and the associated research, ensuring a balanced, comprehensive perspective.

Safety and Precautions

Despite its potential benefits, the Wim Hof Method is not devoid of risks due to its intense nature and involvement of cold exposure, making it unsuitable for some individuals. Those with certain health conditions, notably cardiovascular issues, should exercise caution. Even healthy individuals are advised to begin gradually, ideally under professional supervision. We will unpack these precautions in detail to ensure a safe, beneficial practice.

Conclusion

The Wim Hof Method signifies a bold, exhilarating frontier in the breathwork sphere. Its fusion of controlled breathing, cold exposure, and concentrated meditation offers a distinctive pathway towards enhanced health and vitality. However, as with all advanced breathwork techniques, it necessitates respect, understanding, and appropriate guidance. When these elements are in place, the Wim Hof Method can serve as a formidable tool in your wellness repertoire.

In forthcoming sections, we will continue our deep exploration into the profound realm of breathwork, addressing how to integrate these techniques into daily routines and employ them to meet specific health and wellness objectives.

The Benefits and Best Use Cases for Each Technique

Venturing deeper into the realm of breathwork reveals a fascinating landscape, where not all techniques are equal. Each comes with its unique strengths, tailored to various scenarios. Comprehending the subtle distinctions between these methods can substantially enrich your breathwork practice, enabling a customization that perfectly aligns with your personal needs and goals.

Pranayama Techniques: Balance and Mind-Body Connection

The versatility of Pranayama techniques is truly remarkable. From the energizing and detoxifying capabilities of Kapalabhati, the soothing balance provided by Nadi Shodhana, to the tranquility and focus-enhancing qualities of Bhramari,

Pranayama exercises cater to a range of needs. Regular Pranayama practice fosters a robust mind-body connection, a critical facet of holistic well-being.

Holotropic Breathwork: Self-Discovery and Emotional Release

Holotropic Breathwork serves a distinct purpose. Less focused on physical well-being, it shines a spotlight on psychological and emotional exploration. The practice can help individuals release pent-up emotions, address unresolved trauma, and attain a sense of inner wholeness. However, due to its intense nature, Holotropic Breathwork should be undertaken under the watchful eye of a trained professional.

Wim Hof Method: Resilience and Vitality

In contrast, the Wim Hof Method is about nurturing resilience and vitality. Regular engagement with this practice can potentially boost the immune response, amplify energy levels, and fortify stress resilience. This method is especially beneficial for athletes, adventurers, and those pushing their physical boundaries. However, the method's incorporation of cold exposure necessitates careful preparation.

Comparing the Techniques

While each technique has unique offerings, they also share common threads. All involve conscious breath control, require regular practice for optimal benefits, and serve as tools for enhancing well-being and self-awareness. Choosing among them depends on your individual goals, lifestyle, preferences, and current health status.

Conclusion

Grasping the strengths and most effective use cases for

each advanced breathwork technique equips you to make an informed decision about which methods to integrate into your routine. Importantly, these techniques are not mutually exclusive—you can practice multiple techniques, employing them for different purposes or at varying times. The ultimate goal isn't to master all techniques, but to uncover what best serves you, enhancing your journey towards optimal well-being.

Precautions and Tips for Advanced Practices

Breathwork is largely a safe and beneficial practice. However, when venturing into more advanced techniques, certain precautions become necessary. The power of breathwork lies in its capacity to influence physiological and psychological processes, but this potency also calls for respect and caution. Here, we will guide you on how to safely and responsibly approach advanced breathwork techniques.

Precautions for Advanced Breathwork

While simple breathwork practices are generally safe for everyone, some advanced techniques, owing to their intensity, necessitate careful approach. Techniques like Holotropic Breathwork can evoke potent emotional and psychological experiences, which could prove challenging for some individuals. It's recommended that such practices be carried out under the supervision of trained professionals, and they are not advisable for those with a history of serious mental health issues, cardiovascular diseases, or high blood pressure.

Furthermore, the Wim Hof Method, integrating breathwork with cold exposure, can be system-shocking and must be approached with caution, particularly by those with cardiovascular complications. It's always advisable to consult with a healthcare professional before beginning such practices.

It's important to remember that breathwork should never lead to discomfort or distress. If you experience light-headedness, dizziness, or anxiety during any practice, revert to your normal breathing pattern and seek guidance, if necessary.

Tips for Advanced Practices

Creating a safe and comfortable environment is vital when practicing advanced techniques. Opt for lying down or sitting comfortably in a space where you won't be disturbed. Keeping water within reach is also prudent.

Listen to your body. Although breathwork can be challenging at times, it should never result in physical discomfort. If a technique feels overly taxing, stop and revisit when ready.

Consistency is paramount. Mastery of advanced techniques often demands regular practice. Yet, resist rushing your progress. Allow your body to adapt at its own pace.

Lastly, consider joining a breathwork group or seeking guidance from a trained professional. They can offer invaluable feedback, ensure you're practicing correctly, and provide support through any emerging challenges.

Conclusion

Advanced breathwork techniques can unveil new pathways in your wellness journey. However, they command a higher level of commitment, practice, and caution. By adhering to these precautions and tips, you can safely delve into these powerful practices. Remember, the goal is not to force or hasten progress but to gently guide your body and mind towards deeper states of relaxation, awareness, and self-understanding.

5

Integrating Breathwork into Daily Life

Chapter 5: Integrating Breathwork into Daily Life
The Importance of Consistency

Breathwork, akin to any other practice or skill, relies heavily on consistency for true development. It is not a one-time endeavor, but a transformative journey that deepens over time. It's less about reaching a definitive goal and more about being present throughout the journey. In this segment, we'll discuss the significance of consistency in breathwork and how it engenders profound personal transformation.

Why Consistency Matters

Consistency plays a crucial role in breathwork for several reasons. Firstly, it aids in acquiring the requisite skills to breathe consciously and efficiently. Just as one wouldn't expect to master a musical instrument overnight, breathwork demands consistent practice to foster control, awareness, and the sensitivity needed for advanced techniques.

Secondly, regular breathwork helps to institute new breathing patterns and habits. Many of us have adopted patterns of shallow, rapid breathing due to stress or improper posture. Regular breathwork practice can assist in retraining the body to adopt more advantageous patterns of deep, diaphragmatic breathing, even when not actively practicing.

Lastly, the benefits of breathwork, including stress reduction, mood improvement, and energy enhancement, tend to amplify and sustain with consistent practice. A single session may provide immediate stress or anxiety relief, but regular practice can lead to long-term improvements in mental and physical health.

Establishing a Regular Breathwork Routine

Initiating a regular breathwork routine can be a challenge, particularly when juggling other commitments. Here are some helpful tips to establish and maintain a consistent breathwork practice:

Start Small: Begin with just a few minutes of breathwork daily. Gradually increase session length as comfort and skill level improve.

Schedule Your Practice: Prioritize breathwork by integrating it into your daily schedule, just like any crucial appointment. Consider setting a regular time for practice, such as early morning or late at night.

Create a Comfortable Space: Identify a serene, comfortable space where you won't be disturbed during practice. This could be a specific room, a corner of your bedroom, or even a spot in your backyard.

Vary Your Techniques: To keep your practice intriguing and engaging, alternate between different techniques. This will help you discover which methods work best for you.

Stay Patient and Flexible: If your practice doesn't proceed as planned, that's okay. Some days may be more challenging than others. The key is to remain patient with yourself and flexible in your approach.

Seek Support: If maintaining consistency proves challenging, consider seeking support. This could be through a breathwork group, an online community, or a mentor.

Conclusion

Ultimately, the key to consistency in breathwork, as with any practice, is integration into daily life. It's not about perfection, but progress. Remember that every breath offers an opportunity to practice, whether during formal meditation or while waiting in line at the grocery store. By prioritizing consistency, you will not only enrich your breathwork practice but also enhance your overall well-being.

Building a Daily Breathwork Routine

Incorporating a daily breathwork routine into an already packed schedule might seem intimidating. However, akin to habitual activities like brushing your teeth or making your bed, regular breathwork can become a seamless part of your life over time. With careful planning, tenacity, and a few practical strategies, you can craft a breathwork routine that perfectly complements your lifestyle. In this section, we'll guide you through the process of structuring a daily breathwork routine that is attuned to your personal needs, lifestyle, and goals.

When to Practice

The choice of when to engage in breathwork can significantly influence the consistency and efficacy of your routine. Different times of the day might be more suitable for different individuals, depending on factors such as their daily schedule, energy levels, and personal inclinations. For instance, some may find early morning practice ideal to kick-start the day with positivity, while others might prefer winding down with breathwork in the evening. Try experimenting with various times to discover what suits you best, remembering that consistency is paramount.

Where to Practice

Identifying the right place for your breathwork sessions is equally significant. Choose a tranquil, comfortable, and undisturbed space where you can focus entirely on your breathing without distractions. This could be a designated corner in your home, office, or even a secluded spot in a local park. The more you associate this location with relaxation and mindfulness, the more effective your practice will be.

How to Practice

Crafting a suitable routine involves deciding on the length of your practice and the techniques you employ. If you're just starting, a 5-10 minute session might be sufficient, gradually increasing as you gain comfort and skill. As for the techniques, alternate between a few that you are comfortable with and that cater to your current needs. For instance, if stress is prevalent, calming techniques like box breathing or diaphragmatic breathing might be appropriate. Conversely, if you need to stimulate your body and mind, the Wim Hof Method or Kapalabhati could be advantageous.

Tailoring Your Routine The key to a successful breathwork routine lies in personalization. There's no one-size-fits-all solution; what's most crucial is that your practice aligns with your unique needs, preferences, and lifestyle. This might mean conducting shorter sessions more frequently throughout the day, or dedicating a longer session at a specific time that's most convenient. Listen to your body's responses and adjust your practice as needed.

Conclusion

Establishing a daily breathwork routine is an investment in your wellness. It might necessitate time, patience, and experimentation, but the subsequent benefits—reduced stress, heightened focus, and overall emotional equilibrium—are worth the commitment. Remember, the goal isn't to concoct a flawless routine, but to build a regular practice that you anticipate and that meaningfully contributes to your well-being.

Breathwork for Morning and Evening Routines

The incorporation of breathwork into your daily regimen can drastically enhance your overall well-being. Initiating your day with specific breathwork techniques can set an upbeat and energized mood for the day ahead. Conversely, concluding your day with different techniques can encourage relaxation and facilitate better sleep. This section will delve into how you can strategically employ breathwork to frame your day, laying the groundwork for achievement and tranquility from dawn to dusk.

Breathwork in the Morning

The morning provides a potent opportunity for breathwork. Launching your day with a concentrated breathing routine can invigorate your body, declutter your mind, and establish an optimistic tone for the day ahead. The objective of morning breathwork is to leave you feeling alert, focused, and primed to tackle whatever the day might present.

Several techniques are particularly suitable for morning practice. For instance, the Wim Hof Method, which melds controlled hyperventilation with breath retention, can energize your body and sharpen your focus. Similarly, a technique like Kapalabhati, also known as the 'Skull Shining Breath' in Pranayama tradition, involves a sequence of swift, forceful exhales followed by passive inhales. This can also stimulate the body and mind, equipping you for a productive day.

Breathwork in the Evening

In the evening, your breathwork practice should shift its focus towards relaxation, stress relief, and preparation for sleep. The evening is the ideal time to slow down, release the tensions of the day, and ready your mind and body for restful sleep.

Breathing techniques like Box Breathing, where you inhale, hold, exhale, and hold your breath for equal counts, can help slow down your heart rate and induce a state of calm. Another effective evening technique is the 4-7-8 method, which can function as a natural sedative for the nervous system, easing you into a relaxed state conducive to sleep.

Considerations and Tips

These are general guidelines, and it's important to

remember that everyone is unique. What suits you best may differ from what suits others. Experiment with different techniques at various times of the day to identify what aligns best with your needs.

Conclusion

Incorporating breathwork into your morning and evening routines can substantially enrich your daily life, helping you initiate and conclude your day on a positive note. These mindful breathing moments can act as anchors, grounding you in the present and aiding you in navigating your day with increased serenity, clarity, and intention.

Using Breathwork in Stressful Situations

Stress is an unavoidable aspect of life, but our response to it can significantly influence our overall well-being. Breathwork stands as a readily accessible tool that can be employed anytime, anywhere to help manage stress and restore tranquility. By influencing our autonomic nervous system, breathwork aids in shifting our body from a 'fight or flight' response to a 'rest and digest' state. This section will explore the most effective breathwork techniques for stress management and provide guidance on their application in stressful scenarios.

Understanding Stress

Before diving into specific techniques, it's crucial to comprehend the physiological reactions to stress. When we confront a stressful situation, our sympathetic nervous system springs into action, instigating a series of responses including an increased heart rate, rapid breathing, and heightened alertness. While these reactions are vital for addressing immediate threats, chronic activation can lead to health complications.

Breathwork can help disrupt this stress response, tilting the balance towards the parasympathetic nervous system, responsible for rest and recuperation.

Techniques for Acute Stress

In the throes of a high-stress situation, certain breathwork techniques can swiftly diminish the intensity of your stress response. For instance, Box breathing, with its equal counts of inhaling, holding the breath, exhaling, and holding the breath again, helps slow your breathing rate and soothe your nervous system. Another apt technique for acute stress is the 4-7-8 method, designed by Dr. Andrew Weil. This technique, which incorporates inhaling for 4 counts, holding for 7, and exhaling for 8, is considered a natural sedative for the nervous system.

Techniques for Chronic Stress

To manage chronic stress, a consistent, daily breathwork practice proves more beneficial. Diaphragmatic breathing, also known as belly breathing, is a stellar technique for promoting comprehensive stress reduction. Regular practice of this technique helps retrain your body to breathe more efficiently and respond to stress more calmly. Pranayama techniques like Nadi Shodhana, also known as Alternate Nostril Breathing, are also valuable for managing chronic stress. Regular application of these techniques aids in balancing the nervous system and fostering a sense of calm and clarity.

Considerations and Tips

While breathwork stands as a potent tool for stress management, remember that it's one piece of a comprehensive stress management strategy. Other activities such as regular physical exercise, sufficient sleep, a healthy diet, and social connection are also essential for managing stress effectively.

Conclusion

Breathwork can serve as a potent ally in your stress management toolkit, providing a natural and accessible method to regain calm during stressful situations. By mastering and practicing these techniques, you can cultivate a heightened sense of control over your stress response and navigate life's challenges with greater ease and tranquillity.

Mindful Breathing and Everyday Activities

Though dedicating specific time for breathwork practice is advantageous, it's not the sole method to harness the power of your breath. Blending mindful breathing into your day-to-day activities is another significant way to boost your mindfulness and well-being. It empowers you to remain connected with your breath, maintaining a serene and centered state all day. In this section, we'll discuss strategies to weave mindful breathing into various facets of your life.

Understanding Mindful Breathing

Mindful breathing entails concentrating your attention on the flow of your breath, in and out. It's about being present with each breath, acknowledging the sensations it induces without trying to manipulate or control it. This breathwork type helps root you in the present moment and serves as an anchor to refocus your attention when your mind starts to wander.

Mindful Breathing While Walking

Walking presents an excellent opportunity to practice mindful breathing. Try to synchronize your breath with your steps, perhaps inhaling for three steps and exhaling for the next three. This synchronization can morph a simple walk into a mobile meditation, aiding you in staying centered and present.

Mindful Breathing During Household Chores

Even mundane tasks such as washing dishes, cooking, or cleaning can become avenues for mindful breathing. As you perform these tasks, direct your attention to your breath. Notice how your breath's rhythm correlates with your movements and instills a sense of tranquility and focus on the task at hand.

Mindful Breathing at Work

Work can often be a source of stress and strain. Infusing mindful breathing into your workday can aid in managing stress levels, improving focus, and boosting productivity. Take regular 'breath breaks' throughout the day to check in with your breath and quiet your mind. You can also utilize mindful breathing techniques during meetings or challenging tasks to maintain a state of serene focus.

Mindful Breathing During Exercise

Exercise is another activity that can be enhanced with mindful breathing. Whether you're practicing yoga, lifting weights, or cycling, being conscious of your breath can augment your performance and make your workout more enjoyable. It bridges the mind and body, bringing a sense of unity and presence to your exercise regimen.

Conclusion

By infusing mindful breathing into your everyday activities, you can transform mundane moments into opportunities for mindfulness and tranquility. This practice lets you weave a thread of consciousness throughout your day, cultivating a state of presence that extends beyond your dedicated breathwork or meditation sessions. As you grow more attuned to your breath, you may discover a profound sense of calm and clarity permeating all areas of your life.

Overcoming Challenges in Breathwork Practice

Embarking on a new journey of acquiring breathwork skills can present challenges. These hurdles might include finding time, maintaining focus, or dealing with physical discomfort, making the practice appear daunting. But remember, every obstacle also serves as an opportunity for growth. This section will address these common breathwork practice challenges and provide practical solutions to help you navigate through them.

Finding Time for Practice

One frequent challenge is incorporating breathwork into a hectic schedule. A solution could be to start by dedicating just a few minutes daily to the practice. Early mornings or before bed might provide peaceful moments suitable for breathwork. Alternatively, infuse breathwork into activities you already engage in, like commuting or meal prep. Prioritize consistency over duration; even a few minutes each day can have a significant impact.

Maintaining Focus

In today's world full of distractions, maintaining focus can be a hurdle. If your mind wanders during breathwork, exercise patience. When you notice your attention drifting, gently return your focus to your breath without judgment. Initially, using guided breathwork practices could be beneficial, offering a framework for your focus.

Managing Physical Discomfort

Some individuals might experience physical discomfort like lightheadedness or tingling sensations, especially with intense breathwork techniques. It's crucial to listen to your body's signals. If discomfort arises, ease your practice or revert to normal breathing. As your body adjusts over time, these sensations will likely decrease.

Conclusion

Navigating and overcoming challenges in your breathwork practice is an integral part of the journey. Each breathwork session is unique—some days might feel more effortless than others, which is perfectly okay. The aim is not to achieve perfection but to foster a deeper connection with your breath and yourself. Be patient, continue practicing, and trust the process. Customize these strategies as needed to align with your individual circumstances and needs. As you persevere in overcoming these challenges, you'll find your breathwork practice becoming a more rewarding and transformative aspect of your life.

6

Breathwork for Specific Outcomes

Chapter 6: Breathwork for Specific Outcomes
Breathwork for Stress Management

Stress, a pervasive element of contemporary life, can originate from various sources such as professional pressures, interpersonal challenges, health worries, or the relentless tempo of today's society. While stress represents a natural physiological reaction, chronic exposure can adversely impact our physical and mental health. Breathwork, a mind-body technique, offers a potent mechanism to efficiently manage stress and bolster general wellness.

Our breathing pattern directly influences stress through the autonomic nervous system, comprising two primary branches: the sympathetic nervous system (SNS) – triggering 'fight or flight' responses, and the parasympathetic nervous system (PNS) – initiating 'rest and digest' responses. Stress activates the SNS, resulting in heightened heart rate, blood pressure, and respiratory rate. On the other hand, the PNS, when stimulated through deep, slow breathing, can help diminish these responses, fostering relaxation and stress reduction.

Breathwork Techniques for Stress Management

Various breathwork techniques can significantly aid in managing stress. Here are a few noteworthy ones:

- Box Breathing: This method involving inhaling, holding the breath, exhaling, and again holding the breath for equal durations can help slow the breathing rate, prompt the PNS, and encourage tranquility.
- 4-7-8 Breathing: Created by Dr. Andrew Weil, this technique is akin to a natural tranquilizer for the nervous system. A specific pattern of inhaling for 4 counts, holding for 7, and exhaling for 8 effectively mitigates stress and anxiety.
- Diaphragmatic Breathing: Also known as belly breathing, this technique promotes deeper, more efficient breathing, contributing to enhanced relaxation and stress reduction.

Incorporating Breathwork into Your Routine for Stress Management

To reap the stress-reducing advantages of breathwork, its regular integration into your daily routine is essential. Some recommendations include:

- Morning Practice: Commencing your day with breathwork can set a positive tone. Select a serene, comfortable space for uninterrupted practice. Even a 5-10 minutes session can have a substantial impact.
- Breaks Throughout the Day: Brief breathwork intervals during the day can help manage emerging stress. Merely a few minutes of concentrated breathing can soothe your mind and body.
- Evening Practice: An evening breathwork session can alleviate the day's stress and improve sleep quality. Consider incorporating breathwork into your pre-sleep routine.
- During Stressful Situations: Breathwork can be employed anytime, anywhere. In stressful situations, focusing on your breath for a few moments can restore calmness and clarity.

Conclusion

In our rapid, contemporary world, stress management is vital for preserving health and well-being. Breathwork offers a straightforward yet potent tool for stress management, easily incorporated into daily routines. The appeal of breathwork lies in its accessibility and simplicity; it merely requires a few minutes and your breath.

While the aforementioned techniques are proven effective for stress management, individual responses to breathwork can vary. What works best for one may not suit another as well. Hence, experimenting with different techniques, discovering what suits you best, and exercising patience with yourself is critical.

As you continue practicing, you'll become more familiar with your unique breathing patterns and develop heightened sensitivity to early signs of stress. Over time, breathwork can become your primary stress management tool—a natural, effective method to restore balance, foster relaxation, and enhance overall well-being.

Breathwork for Improved Focus and Productivity

In an era rife with distractions, achieving sustained focus and productivity presents a significant challenge. However, breathwork—the deliberate regulation of your breathing—can be an effective strategy for improving these vital cognitive functions. This potential lies within the intricate relationships between our respiration, nervous system, and mental state.

Breathing is an automatic operation governed by the autonomic nervous system, which also manages various bodily functions such as heart rate and digestion. By consciously controlling our breathing, we can exert influence over our autonomic nervous system, thereby modulating our mental state. For example, certain breathwork techniques can activate the parasympathetic nervous system, which facilitates relaxation and helps declutter the mind. Conversely, other techniques can stimulate the sympathetic nervous system, increasing alertness and focus.

Breathwork Techniques for Improved Focus and Productivity

Several breathwork techniques can notably enhance focus and productivity:

- Box Breathing: This technique incorporates a concentration element by coordinating four parts of the breath, thereby enhancing concentration and calming the mind, facilitating better focus on tasks.
- Kapalabhati (Skull Shining Breath): This invigorating Pranayama technique involves rapid, forceful exhalations followed by passive inhalations. It energizes the body and mind, thereby enhancing alertness and concentration.
- Nadi Shodhana (Alternate Nostril Breathing): This technique involves alternately inhaling and exhaling through one nostril at a time. It is thought to balance the brain's two hemispheres, fostering mental clarity and focus.

Incorporating Breathwork into Your Routine for Improved Focus and Productivity

To harness the focus-enhancing and productivity-boosting benefits of breathwork, its integration into your daily routine is essential. Here are some recommendations:

- Morning Practice: Begin your day with a breathwork session to establish a positive, focused tone. Techniques like Kapalabhati can be particularly energizing.
- Breaks During Work or Study Sessions: Breaks are crucial for maintaining productivity during extended work or study periods. A few minutes of breathwork during these intervals can refresh your mind and sustain focus.
- During Times of Mental Fog or Distraction: If you're

struggling to concentrate or experiencing mental fog, a brief breathwork session can clear your mind and re-energize you. Techniques like Box Breathing or Nadi Shodhana can be especially beneficial.

Conclusion

In today's world, with its numerous distractions and common mental overload, possessing tools to enhance focus and productivity is invaluable. Breathwork is one such tool—a simple yet potent practice that can be incorporated into your daily routine to promote greater clarity, concentration, and productivity.

The effectiveness of breathwork resides in its flexibility and accessibility. You can utilize it whenever you need, whether starting your day with focus and energy, taking a mental break during a hectic workday, or re-centering when you feel overwhelmed or distracted.

Mastering breathwork, like any skill, requires time and practice. Yet, with perseverance, you can tap into the power of your breath to enhance your cognitive performance, transforming your work or study sessions into more productive and enjoyable experiences. The key is to identify the techniques that best suit you and practice them consistently.

Breathwork for Athletic Performance

Athletic performance hinges not merely on physical strength or prowess—it also depends on mental resilience, focus, and efficient physiological functioning. Breathwork, the conscious control of your breathing, can significantly enhance these aspects, making it an indispensable tool for athletes and those engaged in physically intensive activities.

Breathwork can bolster athletic performance in a multitude of ways. It aids in regulating the nervous system, controlling the stress response during high-stakes situations. It can also enhance cardiovascular efficiency and oxygen utilization, which contributes to improved endurance and recovery. Additionally, breathwork enhances focus and mindfulness, enabling athletes to remain in the present moment, perform better under pressure, and learn more effectively from their training experiences.

Breathwork Techniques for Athletic Performance

Several breathwork techniques are particularly beneficial for improving athletic performance:

- Diaphragmatic Breathing: Also known as belly breathing, this technique encourages full oxygen exchange and slows the heartbeat, contributing to improved cardiovascular performance and endurance.
- Box Breathing: This technique involves inhaling, holding the breath, exhaling, and then holding the breath again, assisting with stress management and maintaining focus during high-pressure situations.
- Wim Hof Method: This technique, developed by Dutch extreme athlete Wim Hof, combines specific breathing patterns with cold exposure and meditation. It is claimed to enhance various athletic performance measures, including cardiovascular efficiency, mental focus, and resilience against extreme conditions.

Incorporating Breathwork into Athletic Training and Recovery

Various strategies exist for incorporating breathwork into athletic training and recovery:

- Pre-Training: A breathwork session before training can prime the body and mind for upcoming physical exertion. Techniques like Diaphragmatic Breathing can help optimize cardiovascular function and oxygen supply.
- During Training: Maintaining conscious control of your breath during training sessions can help manage exertion and maintain focus. Techniques like Box Breathing can be particularly effective in managing the stress response during intense or high-pressure moments.
- Post-Training Recovery: After training, breathwork can be utilized to promote recovery and relaxation. Techniques that stimulate the parasympathetic nervous system, like Diaphragmatic Breathing, can help slow the heart rate, promote relaxation, and enhance recovery.

Conclusion

In the realm of sports and physical performance, breathwork can prove to be a powerful asset. By consciously controlling and adjusting our breath, we can directly influence our physiological and mental states, leading to improved performance and recovery.

Breathwork not only boosts physiological functions critical for athletic performance, such as cardiovascular efficiency and oxygen utilization, but it also heightens mental focus and stress management—key elements for performing under pressure.

As an athlete, integrating breathwork into your training and recovery regimen can help you tap into these benefits. Whether it's prepping your body and mind for training, managing your exertion and focus during training, or enhancing your recovery post-training, breathwork can be an invaluable addition to your performance toolkit.

Remember, breathwork is a practice, and its benefits accumulate over time. Regular and consistent practice can lead to more pronounced benefits, transforming not just your athletic performance, but also your overall well-being.

Breathwork for Emotional Release and Healing

In our lives, many of us carry emotional burdens that can manifest as chronic stress, tension, or even physical discomfort. Breathwork, the practice of conscious control over breathing, presents a potent pathway to confront these emotional barriers, promoting healing and emotional well-being. It's a transformative process that utilizes deep, deliberate breathing to influence our mental, emotional, and physical states.

Various traditions and therapeutic practices have long recognized the intricate relationship between breathing and emotions. Emotions are not merely psychological phenomena—they also involve physiological changes, including shifts in our breathing patterns. By consciously manipulating our breath, we can directly influence our emotional state, providing an effective tool for emotional regulation and healing.

Breathwork Techniques for Emotional Release and Healing

Several breathwork techniques have been associated with promoting emotional release and healing:

- Holotropic Breathwork: Developed by psychiatrist Stanislav Grof, this practice involves deep, rapid breathing combined with evocative music to facilitate non-ordinary states of consciousness. It can enable profound emotional release and insights.
- Rebirthing Breathwork: Also known as Conscious Energy Breathing, this technique involves connected, circular breathing (inhaling and exhaling without pausing), which can lead to deep emotional release and healing.
- Pranayama Techniques: Practices like Nadi Shodhana (Alternate Nostril Breathing) and Bhramari (Bee Breathing) can help balance the nervous system, promote calmness, and facilitate emotional processing.

Incorporating Breathwork into Emotional Healing

Incorporating breathwork into a routine for emotional healing requires patience, consistency, and often, guidance from a trained professional. The process can involve:

- Regular Practice: Establishing a regular breathwork practice is crucial. This allows individuals to develop a deeper connection gradually with their breath and emotional landscape.

- Safe Environment: Practicing breathwork in a safe, comfortable space where emotional release can occur uninhibited is essential. This could be at home or in a guided group setting.
- Professional Guidance: Working with a trained professional can provide necessary support, particularly for practices like Holotropic or Rebirthing Breathwork, which can evoke intense emotional experiences.
- Integration: Breathwork is often just one part of an emotional healing journey. It can be used in conjunction with other therapeutic processes, such as psychotherapy, to help process and integrate the emotional experiences and insights that surface.

Conclusion

Breathwork can be a transformative tool for emotional release and healing, offering a route to access and process emotions that might otherwise remain unacknowledged. It helps foster a deeper connection with our inner emotional landscape, promoting self-awareness, self-understanding, and ultimately, self-healing.

However, it's essential to approach breathwork for emotional healing with care, particularly when dealing with traumatic or deeply buried emotions. Guidance from a trained professional is highly recommended.

Remember, emotional healing is a journey that takes time and patience. Each breathwork session represents a step along this path, helping to gradually release emotional burdens and move towards greater emotional well-being and personal growth.

Breathwork for Meditation and Spiritual Growth

In many cultures and spiritual traditions across the globe, breath is considered a vital bridge, interconnecting the body, mind, and spirit. The conscious control of breath, or breathwork, can lead to profound states of consciousness and significantly enhance the meditative experience. This exploration delves into the intricate connection between breathwork, meditation, and spiritual growth. It offers valuable techniques to deepen meditation practices and heighten spiritual awareness.

The Role of Breath in Meditation

Breath occupies a central position in most forms of meditation. It operates as a focal point, consistently bringing our attention back to the immediacy of the present moment each time the mind strays. Employing specific breathing techniques can induce tranquility in the mind and body, thus preparing them for deeper states of meditation. Moreover, certain breathing patterns can induce altered states of consciousness, thereby providing deeper insights and experiences of a spiritual nature.

Breathwork Techniques for Meditation and Spiritual Growth

Several breathwork techniques can be particularly conducive to meditation and spiritual growth:

- Anapana: This practice involves mindfully observing

natural breath as taught in Vipassana meditation. It serves to enhance mindfulness and self-awareness.

- Nadi Shodhana (Alternate Nostril Breathing): This pranayama technique balances the body's energy systems and is believed to harmonize the two hemispheres of the brain, thus inducing a sense of peace and clarity that is ideal for meditation.
- Sudarshan Kriya: This rhythmic breathing technique, developed by The Art of Living foundation, reportedly has profound effects on mental and emotional states, leading to increased clarity, calmness, and joy.
- Holotropic Breathwork: While this technique is often used for psychological healing, its ability to induce non-ordinary states of consciousness can lead to profound spiritual experiences.

Incorporating Breathwork into Spiritual Practices

Integrating breathwork into your spiritual practice may involve using a specific technique as a precursor to meditation. For instance, Nadi Shodhana can be employed to soothe the mind and balance energy before engaging in silent meditation. For some, breathwork itself may constitute the spiritual practice. This is the case with Holotropic Breathwork, where the altered state of consciousness induced by the breathing pattern facilitates deep spiritual exploration.

Conclusion

Breathwork and meditation are interwoven practices, each amplifying the effect of the other. Consistent practice of breathwork can profoundly deepen your meditation, enhancing your capacity for self-awareness, and potentially facilitating profound spiritual experiences. It is always essential that your breathwork practice be tailored to suit your specific needs, preferences, and spiritual objectives. As you traverse the landscape of your breath, you may just find yourself exploring the contours of your own spirit.

Personalizing Your Breathwork Practice

Breathwork is an inherently personal journey, with its effectiveness dependent on an individual's unique needs, aspirations, and preferences. The variety of breathwork techniques we've examined can serve as a comprehensive toolbox, providing you the freedom to select, amalgamate, and modify methods to perfectly align with your lifestyle and goals. This chapter offers guidance on how you can tailor your breathwork practice to your personal needs.

Identifying Your Objectives

The primary step towards personalizing your breathwork practice lies in identifying your goals. Are you seeking stress management, enhancement of athletic performance, deepening of your meditation, or support for emotional healing? Comprehending what you aim to achieve from breathwork will steer you towards the most fitting techniques.

Choosing Techniques

Once your objectives are clear, you can begin to select techniques that align with them. For example, if your aim is to alleviate stress, calming techniques such as Box Breathing or 4-7-8 Breathing may be ideal. If enhancing your meditation practice is your goal, techniques such as Anapana or Nadi Shodhana might be more appropriate.

Adapting and Combining Techniques

Do not feel limited by the provided guidelines for each technique—feel free to adapt them as per your comfort. You might discover that slightly adjusting the breath ratios in a technique makes it more beneficial for you. Additionally, do not hesitate to combine techniques to meet your individual needs.

Creating a Routine

Consistency is a vital element in breathwork. Develop a routine that seamlessly fits into your schedule—whether it's a morning practice to kick-start your day, a midday session for stress relief, or an evening ritual to unwind.

Conclusion

Remember, your journey with breathwork should be one of exploration and self-discovery. Take your time, listen to your body, and make necessary adjustments along the way. With patience and perseverance, you will discover the ideal blend of techniques that resonate with you, promoting health, well-being, and inner growth.

7

Understanding Your Breath: Physiology and Neuroscience

Chapter 7: Understanding Your Breath: Physiology and Neuroscience

The Mechanics of Breathing

Breathwork is an inherently personal journey, with its effectiveness dependent on an individual's unique needs, aspirations, and preferences. The variety of breathwork techniques we've examined can serve as a comprehensive toolbox, providing you the freedom to select, amalgamate, and modify methods to perfectly align with your lifestyle and goals. This chapter offers guidance on how you can tailor your breathwork practice to your personal needs.

Identifying Your Objectives

The primary step towards personalizing your breathwork practice lies in identifying your goals. Are you seeking stress management, enhancement of athletic performance, deepening of your meditation, or support for emotional healing? Comprehending what you aim to achieve from breathwork will steer you towards the most fitting techniques.

Choosing Techniques

Once your objectives are clear, you can begin to select techniques that align with them. For example, if your aim is to alleviate stress, calming techniques such as Box Breathing or 4-7-8 Breathing may be ideal. If enhancing your meditation practice is your goal, techniques such as Anapana or Nadi Shodhana might be more appropriate.

Adapting and Combining Techniques

Do not feel limited by the provided guidelines for each technique—feel free to adapt them as per your comfort. You might discover that slightly adjusting the breath ratios in a technique makes it more beneficial for you. Additionally, do not hesitate to combine techniques to meet your individual needs.

Creating a Routine

Consistency is a vital element in breathwork. Develop a routine that seamlessly fits into your schedule—whether it's a morning practice to kick-start your day, a midday session for stress relief, or an evening ritual to unwind.

Conclusion

Remember, your journey with breathwork should be one of exploration and self-discovery. Take your time, listen to your body, and make necessary adjustments along the way. With patience and perseverance, you will discover the ideal blend of techniques that resonate with you, promoting health, well-being, and inner growth.

The Autonomic Nervous System and Breath

Breathing acts as a unique interface between the conscious and unconscious realms of our mind. While it operates automatically, under the control of the autonomic nervous system (ANS), it can also be consciously manipulated. This distinct characteristic allows breathwork to be a powerful means to influence the ANS and, consequently, our physiological and emotional states. To grasp this connection, we must explore the architecture of the ANS, especially its sympathetic and parasympathetic divisions, and understand their relationship with our breath.

Overview of the Autonomic Nervous System

The ANS is a subdivision of our nervous system that regulates many of our body's involuntary functions, such as heart rate, digestion, and respiratory rate. It is primarily bifurcated into the sympathetic nervous system (SNS) and the parasympathetic nervous system (PNS).

The Sympathetic Nervous System and the 'Fight or Flight' Response

The SNS primes the body for immediate action. It instigates the 'fight or flight' response in the face of a perceived threat, increasing heart and breath rates, dilating pupils, and raising blood pressure to prepare the body for combat or escape.

The Parasympathetic Nervous System and the 'Rest and Digest' Response

In contrast, the PNS activates the body's 'rest and digest'

functions. It is most dominant during periods of rest and relaxation, aiding in slowing the heart rate, reducing blood pressure, stimulating digestion, and fostering a slower, more profound breathing pattern.

The Role of Breathwork in Influencing the ANS

Breathwork can be utilized as a switch to toggle the balance between the SNS and PNS. Rapid, shallow breathing can stimulate the SNS, promoting alertness and energy. Conversely, slow, deep breathing can bolster PNS activity, fostering relaxation and tranquility. Understanding this mechanism can empower us to strategically employ breathwork to induce desired states of arousal or relaxation.

Conclusion

The interaction between breath and the ANS underscores the potency of breathwork. By intentionally altering our breathing patterns, we can manipulate our ANS and adjust our physical and mental states. This principle forms the bedrock of many breathwork practices, highlighting the potential of breathwork as an instrument for self-regulation and overall well-being.

The Autonomic Nervous System and Breath

Breathing is a remarkable process that acts as an intersection between our conscious and unconscious mind. While it primarily functions automatically, orchestrated by the autonomic nervous system (ANS), we also have the ability to control it consciously. This unique dual functionality allows breathwork to serve as a potent tool to influence the ANS, and thus our physiological and emotional states. To comprehend this, it's necessary to delve into the architecture of the ANS, specifically focusing on its sympathetic and parasympathetic divisions, and understand their interaction with our breath.

Overview of the Autonomic Nervous System

The ANS is a subsystem of our nervous system that manages a plethora of the body's automatic functions such as heart rate, digestion, and respiratory rate, among others. It bifurcates into two primary branches: the sympathetic nervous system (SNS) and the parasympathetic nervous system (PNS).

The Sympathetic Nervous System and the 'Fight or Flight' Response

The SNS readies the body for immediate action. It instigates the 'fight or flight' response when we face a perceived threat, heightening heart rate and blood pressure, dilating pupils, and accelerating breath rate to prepare the body to deal with or escape from the danger.

The Parasympathetic Nervous System and the 'Rest and Digest' Response

Contrarily, the PNS initiates the body's 'rest and digest' functions. It is predominantly active during periods of rest and relaxation, assisting in slowing the heart rate, reducing blood pressure, and stimulating digestion. The PNS also fosters a slower and deeper breathing pattern.

The Role of Breathwork in Influencing the ANS

Breathwork can act as a lever to tilt the balance between the SNS and PNS. Fast, shallow breathing can stimulate the SNS, encouraging alertness and energy. On the contrary, slow, deep breathing can bolster PNS activity, fostering relaxation and tranquility. This understanding can aid us in using breathwork strategically to induce desired states of arousal or relaxation.

Conclusion

The intricate interplay between breath and the ANS highlights the power of breathwork. By consciously altering our breathing patterns, we can manipulate our ANS and adjust our physical and mental states. This idea forms the core of numerous breathwork practices and emphasizes the potential of breathwork as an instrument for self-regulation and health enhancement.

The Role of Carbon Dioxide in Breathwork

Breathing, for most of us, brings to mind the essential gas oxygen that is integral to life. However, carbon dioxide (CO_2), often dismissed as a mere waste product destined for exhalation, holds a significant position in our physiological operations. It's crucial to delve into the importance of CO_2, its intricate relationship with our body functions, and how strategically manipulating CO_2 levels via breathwork can lead to significant impacts on our health and consciousness.

Understanding CO2 and Its Role in Respiration

CO_2, the end-product of cellular respiration, plays a critical role in maintaining the pH balance of our body. It combines with water in our bloodstream to form carbonic acid, a compound that disassociates to generate bicarbonate...

CO2 and the Bohr Effect

The Bohr effect, attributed to Danish physiologist Christian Bohr, explains how the oxygen-carrying capacity of our blood fluctuates in response to CO_2 and pH levels. Essentially, heightened CO_2 levels and a reduced pH (more acidic environment) result in a more efficient offloading of oxygen from hemoglobin in our tissues.

Breathwork Techniques and CO2 Manipulation

Various breathwork techniques maneuver our body's CO2 levels in distinct ways. Techniques that involve breath-holding or intentionally slowing down your breathing can escalate CO2 levels, thereby inducing several physiological responses. Conversely, other techniques involving rapid, deep breathing might temporarily decrease CO2 levels.

Safety Considerations

While adjusting CO2 levels through breathwork can elicit a range of effects, it's paramount to practice these techniques safely. Sudden alterations in CO2 can trigger sensations of lightheadedness, dizziness, or even fainting in some instances.

Conclusion

Far from being a simple waste product, CO2 is a vital component of our respiratory physiology. By comprehending and utilizing its role via breathwork, we can exert influence over our health, well being, and state of consciousness in substantial ways. As potent as these practices are, they should always be approached with safety as the paramount concern.

The Impact of Breath on Emotions

Breathing and emotions are deeply interwoven, influencing each other in remarkable ways. Have you noticed when fear or anxiety takes hold, your breath tends to speed up and shallow? Conversely, when you are at peace or joyous, your breathing becomes slow and deep. This section will dissect this intricate connection, explaining the science behind this interplay and illustrating how conscious breath control can empower us to traverse our emotional terrain.

Understanding the Breath-Emotion Connection

Our breathing patterns transform in response to our emotional states. This change in breath can ignite physiological responses that further amplify these emotions. While this cycle can be advantageous when reacting to threats, it can prove detrimental when these responses become chronic.

Impact of Emotional States on Breathing

Various emotions correspond to unique breathing patterns. Anxiety, for example, often results in rapid, shallow breaths, whereas sadness may manifest in sighs. We'll delve into an array of emotions and their associated breathing patterns.

Changing Emotions through Breathwork

Just as our emotions can shape our breathing patterns, conscious breath control can also influence our emotional state. Several breathwork techniques can encourage relaxation, diminish anxiety, promote a sense of joy, or even instigate emotional release. We'll inspect these techniques and their emotional implications in detail.

Scientific Evidence and Further Studies

An expanding body of research underscores the connection between breathing and emotions. Studies have demonstrated that breathwork can positively impact mental health, reducing symptoms of anxiety and depression.

Conclusion

Comprehending the relationship between breathing and emotions unveils a potent tool for emotional self-regulation.

By learning to adjust our breath, we can influence our emotional state, promoting enhanced emotional resilience and well being. As we embark on the exploration of these techniques, remember to approach them with patience and gentleness. Each breath is a step forward on your journey of emotional understanding and growth.

The Breath-Brain Connection

Breathing is intimately tied to the functioning of our brain. It not only delivers the oxygen essential for optimal brain function but also has profound influences on our brainwaves, consciousness, and cognitive abilities. In this section, we will uncover the fascinating connection between breath and brain, highlighting how breathwork can significantly impact our mental state and cognitive performance.

Breath, Brainwaves, and States of Consciousness

Our brain operates on varying frequencies, referred to as brainwaves, which are associated with different states of consciousness. Breathwork can manipulate these brainwaves, assisting in the induction of relaxation, focus, or heightened awareness states.

Breathing and Cognitive Function

Beyond its effects on our mental state, breathing also influences our cognitive functions like attention, memory, and decision-making. Gaining insight into how our breath impacts these cognitive abilities can equip us with powerful tools to enhance our mental performance.

Neuroscience of the Breath-Brain Connection

The field of neuroscience has started to unveil the

mechanisms underlying the breath-brain connection. These include the role of the brainstem, the vagus nerve, and various neurotransmitters. This segment will give a concise overview of our current scientific comprehension of these mechanisms.

Conclusion

The intricate connection between breath and brain highlights the immense power of breathwork. It not only serves as a tool for stress management or energy boost, but it also holds the potential to improve cognitive abilities and alter states of consciousness. If you aim to hone your focus, enhance memory, or deepen your meditation practice, understanding and utilizing the breath-brain connection can be a powerful ally in your journey.

Future Research and the Frontiers of Breathwork

Although our understanding of breathwork has made remarkable progress, there is still much to uncover. Ongoing research continually provides new insights into the physiological, psychological, and spiritual facets of breathwork, making this a thrilling era for enthusiasts in this field. This concluding section will sketch the promising areas for future research and possible advancements in the realm of breathwork.

Current State of Research

In this segment, we will survey existing research findings and their limitations. Despite substantial proof endorsing the benefits of breathwork, numerous studies still have methodological constraints that future research needs to rectify.

Areas for Future Research

Numerous queries about breathwork remain unresolved. For example, how does breathwork influence long-term mental health? Can it be employed to cure specific physical conditions? What are the exact mechanisms through which breathwork affects the brain? This section will probe these and other intriguing queries, suggesting areas where additional research could provide thrilling revelations.

Potential Future Developments

Looking forward, breathwork is expected to be increasingly incorporated into healthcare, athletic training, mental health treatment, and everyday wellness practices. It could also be a key component in technological innovations such as apps and devices crafted to guide and enhance breathwork practices.

Conclusion

Despite the existing uncertainties and unknowns, one fact is undeniable: breathwork possesses tremendous potential. As research progresses and awareness expands, the reputation of breathwork as an accessible, effective, and empowering practice is set to grow further. The future of breathwork is as promising as the practice itself. This marks the end of our exploration into the science of breathwork. Comprehending these principles can fortify your practice and deepen your appreciation of this potent self-care tool. As with all sections, this draft can be modified to better resonate with your expertise and viewpoint.

Addressing Common Misconceptions about Breathwork

Chapter 8: Addressing Common Misconceptions about Breathwork

Misconception: Breathwork is a New-Age Fad

The escalating popularity of breathwork, particularly within wellness and self-help circles, has led some skeptics to label it as a new-age fad. This perception, however, overlooks the historical depth and cultural diversity of breathwork practices. In this section, we aim to debunk the notion of breathwork as a contemporary trend by delving into its historical and cultural origins.

The Ancient Origins of Breathwork

Breathwork has a rich and varied history dating back to ancient civilizations. Practices such as pranayama in yoga from ancient India and Tummo breathing techniques in Tibetan

Buddhism underline the long-standing importance of breath control. In this segment, we will explore these and other early forms of breathwork and their cultural significance.

Breathwork Across Cultures

Breathwork isn't restricted to a single tradition or culture. Instead, it is a globally recognized practice appearing in various forms across societies. This universality underscores the importance assigned to controlled breathing for health, well-being, and spiritual growth across human cultures.

Modern Applications of Ancient Wisdom

The breathwork techniques that are in vogue today often draw upon these ancient practices, merging age-old wisdom with contemporary scientific insights. We will discuss popular modern breathwork techniques, their origins, and how they demonstrate continuity from historical practices to present-day applications.

Conclusion

Far from being a new-age trend, breathwork is a practice deeply rooted in human history, drawing from the wisdom of various cultures and traditions. Contemporary practitioners are following in the footsteps of countless predecessors who have explored the transformative power of breath over centuries. Recognizing this historical context can enhance our appreciation for breathwork and its significant role in human health and spiritual growth.

Misconception: More Oxygen is Always Better

Life as we know it is profoundly dependent on oxygen. It fuels our cells, energizes our bodies, and underpins a host of vital physiological processes. However, the widespread belief that "more oxygen is always better" is a misguided notion. Fundamentally, respiration is a delicate dance between oxygen and carbon dioxide, and any imbalance can lead to harmful consequences. In this section, we aim to debunk the 'more oxygen is better' myth and illuminate the importance of maintaining an optimal respiratory balance.

The Role of Oxygen in the Body

Oxygen's role in our body is undeniably critical, primarily manifesting in cellular respiration where it enables energy production. This segment will provide a comprehensive look at this process, discussing the body's varying oxygen demands under different circumstances and conditions.

The Importance of Carbon Dioxide

Often relegated to the status of a mere waste product, carbon dioxide performs several crucial functions within our bodies. These include maintaining blood pH balance and aiding oxygen delivery to our tissues. This part of the section delves into the role of carbon dioxide, emphasizing why a careful equilibrium between oxygen and carbon dioxide is vital.

The Dangers of Over-Oxygenation

Counter to common intuition, an excessive intake of oxygen can be detrimental, leading to conditions such as hyperventilation and oxygen toxicity. We will discuss these conditions, their causes, and how they impact our bodies.

The Role of Breathwork in Maintaining Respiratory Balance

Breathwork techniques offer an effective way to preserve a healthy balance of oxygen and carbon dioxide, essential for our overall well-being. This portion will explore specific breathwork practices designed to promote balanced respiration.

Conclusion

While oxygen remains a critical element for life, the 'more is better' maxim doesn't hold true in this context. A balanced respiratory system, characterized by adequate levels of both oxygen and carbon dioxide, is a cornerstone of optimal health. Through breathwork, we can learn to regulate our breathing to support this balance, thereby dispelling the myth that more oxygen is always beneficial.

Misconception: Faster, Deeper Breathing is Ideal

There is a prevalent misconception about breathing that faster and deeper breaths are universally beneficial. While such a breathing pattern may be advantageous under certain circumstances, sustained over time, it can lead to hyperventilation and upset the body's balance of oxygen and carbon dioxide. In this section, we aim to dispel this myth and shed light on the advantages of slower, more controlled, and mindful breathing.

The Physiology of Fast, Deep Breathing

Fast, deep breathing, also known as hyperventilation, can trigger various physiological responses. These may include lightheadedness, a tingling sensation, and in severe cases, even fainting. These occur due to excessive breathing which lowers the concentration of carbon dioxide in the blood, leading to a state called respiratory alkalosis. We'll explore this process in depth, outlining how it impacts the body.

The Benefits of Slow, Controlled Breathing

Contrarily, slower, more controlled breathing yields

numerous benefits. It activates the parasympathetic nervous system, ushering in a state of relaxation and calm. Additionally, it helps maintain a healthy balance of oxygen and carbon dioxide within the body. We will examine the science behind these advantages, providing evidence from relevant research studies.

Hyperventilation and Breathwork Practices

Some breathwork techniques do involve controlled hyperventilation, but these practices are typically complemented by breath retention or other strategies to restore balance. Also, they are generally conducted in a controlled, safe environment, often under the supervision of a trained professional. We will discuss hyperventilation's role within these practices and how they steer clear of the pitfalls of unregulated, persistent hyperventilation.

The Role of Mindful Breathing

Mindful breathing, focusing on the rhythm, depth, and quality of breath, amplifies the benefits of slow, controlled breathing, bolstering both physical and mental health. We will explore the concept of mindful breathing and how it can be fostered through breathwork.

Conclusion

While faster, deeper breaths may have their place in certain breathwork techniques or high-stress scenarios, it is not the optimal breathing pattern for everyday life. Slower, controlled, and mindful breathing promotes a healthier balance of oxygen and carbon dioxide, fosters relaxation, and enhances overall well-being. This understanding helps debunk the myth that faster and deeper breathing is invariably the best approach.

Misconception: Breathwork Can Substitute for Medical Treatment

Breathwork is a potent tool for enhancing well-being, managing stress, and supporting overall health. However, a common misunderstanding is that breathwork can supplant medical treatment for serious health conditions. While breathwork can indeed complement medical interventions, it's crucial to comprehend that it should not substitute professional medical advice and treatment.

Breathwork and Its Benefits

We will discuss the myriad potential benefits of breathwork, ranging from stress reduction to enhanced respiratory function. Importantly, we must remember that these benefits bolster general health and well-being and are not intended to treat specific medical conditions.

The Role of Medical Treatment

Medical treatment—be it medication, surgical procedures, or other interventions—is designed to treat specific health conditions and is backed by extensive research and clinical trials. We will delve into the importance of these treatments, highlighting the fundamental differences between medical interventions and breathwork and other complementary practices.

Breathwork as a Complementary Practice

Breathwork can be an invaluable addition to medical treatments. It can help manage side effects, bolster mental health, and amplify the body's inherent healing abilities. We will discuss how breathwork can be integrated into a comprehensive health strategy under the supervision of healthcare professionals.

The Dangers of Forgoing Medical Treatment

Choosing to ignore medical treatment in favor of breathwork can lead to severe, even life-threatening, outcomes. It's vital to seek and adhere to professional medical advice when dealing with health concerns, especially serious conditions. We will tackle the potential risks of neglecting medical treatment and underscore why breathwork should not replace professional healthcare.

Conclusion While breathwork has many benefits and can bolster overall health and well-being, it's vital to understand its limitations. Breathwork should never be used as a replacement for professional medical treatment, particularly for serious health conditions. When used judiciously and appropriately, breathwork can complement medical care, supporting healing and health promotion. This understanding can empower you to make informed decisions about your health and wellness.

Misconception: Breathwork is Always Safe and Suitable for Everyone

Breathwork practices, when approached mindfully and responsibly, are typically safe. However, there is a misconception that all forms of breathwork are universally suitable, irrespective of an individual's health status or conditions. In reality, while breathwork can yield substantial benefits, it may not be appropriate for everyone. Moreover, certain advanced techniques might pose risks if performed incorrectly or without proper supervision.

Understanding Breathwork and Its Effects

We'll delve into the various types of breathwork and their impact on the body and mind. We'll emphasize that the effects can greatly vary based on the specific technique used and the individual practicing it.

Potential Risks and Precautions

This section will explore the potential risks associated with breathwork, particularly the more intense techniques. Topics will include temporary discomfort, the risk of hyperventilation, and the possibility of emotional overwhelm. We will underscore the importance of taking precautions, such as practicing in a safe environment and gradually introducing new techniques.

The Importance of Professional Guidance

Professional guidance can be invaluable, especially when beginning a new breathwork practice or attempting more advanced techniques. We'll investigate the role of trained practitioners and the benefits of seeking their guidance.

Who Should Be Cautious?

Certain individuals, especially those with cardiovascular diseases, respiratory conditions, psychiatric disorders, or pregnant women, should consult with a healthcare provider before embarking on a breathwork practice. We'll discuss why this is vital and the potential risks involved for these individuals.

Conclusion

While breathwork can serve as a powerful tool for self-regulation and wellness, it must be approached with respect and a thorough understanding of its nature. Not all practices are suitable for everyone, and some may carry inherent risks. It's crucial to always take precautions, seek professional guidance when necessary, and consult with a healthcare provider if you have any health concerns. When used wisely, breathwork can significantly contribute to your wellness toolbox.

How to Approach Breathwork with a Balanced Perspective

Breathwork, while a potent practice, only reveals its full potential when used appropriately. Achieving this requires a balanced and discerning mindset, patience, and consistency. In this final section, we will underscore the importance of these attributes and provide guidance on how to cultivate them.

Value of Personal Experience

Breathwork is a highly individual practice, and its effects can vary significantly from person to person. We'll emphasize the value of self-awareness and honoring your unique experiences with different techniques. Understanding and respecting your individual responses is a crucial part of your breathwork journey.

The Role of Consistency

Consistency is key in breathwork, much like physical exercise or learning a new skill. Regular practice enhances your familiarity with the techniques, helping you to embed these habits more deeply, refine your skills, and maximize the benefits over time.

Patience and Breathwork

Breathwork is not a shortcut to wellness but a practice that evolves and deepens over time. We'll stress the importance of patience and understanding, showing how respecting your personal pace can significantly enhance your breathwork experience and result in more profound and lasting changes.

Conclusion In conclusion, it's essential to remember that breathwork is a journey rather than a destination. Approach it with an open mind, value your personal experiences, remain consistent in your practice, and above all, be patient with yourself. With these guiding principles, breathwork can become a deeply rewarding component of your wellness journey.

The Relationship Between Breathwork and Other Wellness Practices

Chapter 9: The Relationship Between Breathwork and Other Wellness Practices

Breathwork and Meditation: Two Sides of the Same Coin

Breathwork and meditation, while unique practices, share commonalities. Both foster mindfulness, alleviate stress, and promote holistic well-being. Each focuses on inward attention, fostering increased internal awareness. Breathwork, by utilizing the powerful force of respiration, provides an anchor for concentration and can thus enhance the depth of meditation. In turn, the increased focus and mindfulness gained through meditation can enrich breathwork, making it a more potent and insightful practice.

Understanding the Interplay

The symbiosis between breathwork and meditation is seen in their shared ability to influence our nervous system and modify our state of mind. Both modalities offer a shift from a 'doing' mode to a 'being' mode where thoughts, emotions, and physical sensations are observed without judgment. Engaging in breathwork can ease the transition into a meditative state, with the continuous rhythm of the breath acting as a grounding force, tethering us to the present moment.

Enhancing Meditation with Breathwork

For those who find meditation challenging, breathwork can be a helpful aid. The active process of breathwork provides the mind a tangible point of focus, reducing distractions and quietening internal dialogue. Initiating a meditation session with a brief period of breathwork can help to soothe the mind, prepare the body, and create an optimal environment for more profound and focused meditation. Techniques such as box breathing or coherent breathing can be particularly beneficial in this context.

Integrating Breathwork into Your Meditation Practice

To merge breathwork into your meditation practice, begin by establishing a comfortable posture and engage in your selected breathwork technique for a few minutes. As your breathing pattern becomes calm and steady, shift your attention to observing the natural rhythm of your breath without trying to manipulate it. Cultivate a mindset of open, nonjudgmental awareness. The goal is not to eliminate thoughts or attain a particular state but to be wholly present with whatever transpires. Whether you're a novice or seasoned mediator, integrating breathwork can add new dimensions to your meditation practice.

The combination of breathwork and meditation can foster a profound sense of tranquility, heighten self-awareness, and bolster capabilities for managing stress and maintaining internal equilibrium. As you navigate this crossroads of breathwork and meditation, remember that everyone's journey is unique. The key is to heed your body and mind's cues and discover what approach resonates best with you.

Breathwork and Yoga: Historical Roots and Shared Principles

Yoga and breathwork both hail from the rich heritage of ancient Indian traditions, underpinned by shared principles. These practices champion mindfulness, presence, and an inner connection. Both cultivate balance, whether between effort and ease in a yoga asana, or through rhythmic modulation of breathing. Within the yoga tradition, breathwork, also known as "pranayama," is considered one of the eight limbs of yoga, underlining its integral role in this discipline.

The Role of Breath in Yoga

The breath holds an essential role within yoga, acting as a bridge linking the body and mind. The rhythm of the breath can guide the choreography of yoga movements. Many yoga instructors guide their students to move "with the breath," pairing inhalations and exhalations with specific actions. The breath also functions as an indicator of exertion—if it becomes strained or irregular, it may signal the need to ease the intensity of a pose. Further, certain pranayama techniques serve to ready the body and mind for meditation, thereby reinforcing the link between breathwork and meditation, as highlighted previously.

Understanding Pranayama

Pranayama is a Sanskrit term composed of 'prana,' referring to the life force or vital energy (commonly equated with breath), and 'ayama,' meaning control or extension. Thus, pranayama involves manipulating or extending the breath to influence this internal life force. Various pranayama techniques yield different impacts—some are calming (like Nadi Shodhana or alternate nostril breathing), while others are energizing (like Kapalabhati or skull shining breath). Familiarizing oneself with these techniques and their impacts can enhance both your yoga and breathwork practices.

Integrating Breathwork and Yoga

Integrating breathwork into yoga practice can be a seamless process. For instance, a yoga session might commence with a few minutes of calming pranayama to quiet the mind, or conclude with an energizing pranayama to invigorate the body. During the asana (pose) practice, mindful breathing can augment the depth and effectiveness of the poses, improve balance and stability, and foster a more mindful, present practice.

In summary, yoga and breathwork are complementary practices that, when synergized, can result in increased physical and mental harmony. Exploring the intersection of these disciplines can enrich your overall wellness journey, offering a more holistic comprehension of these ancient traditions.

Breathwork and Mindfulness

Defining Mindfulness

Mindfulness entails maintaining a moment-by-moment awareness of our thoughts, feelings, bodily sensations, and surrounding environment in a non-judgmental manner. It's about acceptance, meaning we pay attention to our thoughts and feelings without labeling them as good or bad, without trying to suppress or deny them. Rooted in Buddhism, mindfulness has entered the mainstream in recent years, thanks to its practical benefits such as stress reduction, improved focus, increased emotional resilience, and overall mental well being. We will delve deeper into the concept of mindfulness, its historical context, and potential benefits.

The Role of Breath in Fostering Mindfulness

The breath is an invaluable tool in developing mindfulness. Given its ever-present nature, it serves as a stable anchor to the present moment, helping to pacify the mind and reduce mental noise. In addition, the breath mirrors our emotional and physiological states, providing us real-time feedback about our current state of being. Observing the breath, therefore, can become a potent practice of cultivating a mindful presence.

Enhancing Mindfulness with Breathwork

Breathwork can augment mindfulness by offering a tangible focal point for the mind, minimizing distractions, and fostering a sense of calm and clarity. The practice of controlling and modulating the breath can amplify our awareness of the connections between the mind and body, thereby nurturing a deeper sense of mindfulness. Certain breathwork techniques, like mindful breathing or the 4-7-8 technique, can be particularly beneficial in fostering mindfulness.

Practical Tips for Using Breathwork to Cultivate Mindfulness

To utilize breathwork to augment mindfulness, start by designating a regular time slot each day for your breathwork practice. Initiate your session by spending a few moments observing your natural breath, without any intention to control or modify it. Once you have established a clear sense of your innate breathing rhythm, you can begin your selected breathwork technique, maintaining a gentle, non-judgmental awareness of each inhalation and exhalation. After completing your breathwork session, spend a few moments noting any changes in your mental or physical state before transitioning out of your practice.

Incorporating breathwork into your mindfulness regimen can boost your capacity to stay present, manage stress more effectively, and contribute to overall well being. Always remember, your personal experiences and understanding should inform your practice. Tailor these suggested approaches to suit your needs or those of your audience.

Breathwork and Physical Exercise

Understanding the Physiology of Breath and Exercise

During physical exertion, our body's demand for oxygen increases and so does the need to expel carbon dioxide, a byproduct of energy metabolism. This physiological demand necessitates effective and efficient breathing. Breathing is not just an automatic function; it can be voluntarily controlled and optimized. When we breathe improperly or inefficiently, it limits our ability to meet the oxygen demand, potentially affecting athletic performance. This section delves into the physiology of breath during exercise, discussing how effective breathing supports physical exertion and the ramifications for athletic performance.

Breathwork for Athletic Performance

Various breathwork techniques have the potential to boost athletic performance by enhancing oxygen efficiency, improving endurance, and facilitating recovery. Techniques such as "pursed-lip breathing" or "diaphragmatic breathing" aid athletes in using oxygen more effectively. Other techniques like "box breathing" or "4-7-8 breathing" can foster relaxation and expedite recovery post intense physical exertion. We will delve into these techniques, discussing their potential benefits and providing guidance on how to incorporate them into an athletic routine.

Science Behind Breathwork and Exercise

Recent scientific research has highlighted the relationship between breathwork and athletic performance. Studies have shown that techniques such as diaphragmatic breathing can enhance sports performance by boosting oxygen intake and reducing heart rate. Furthermore, breath-holding practices can stimulate the body's adaptive response, improving our capacity to utilize oxygen and increasing our tolerance to carbon dioxide. This section will review these studies, providing evidence-based insights into the benefits of integrating breathwork into your fitness routine.

Incorporating Breathwork Into Your Workout Routine

There are several practical ways to incorporate breathwork into your workout routine. You might begin your workout with a few minutes of calming breathwork to center your focus and prepare your body for the impending physical exertion. During the workout, conscious control of your breathing can enhance performance, especially during high-intensity periods. Following your workout, a few minutes of relaxing breathwork can help transition your body back to its resting state and aid in recovery.

Remember, everyone's body and athletic needs are unique. What works best may differ from person to person. Hence, it's essential to experiment with different techniques, listen to your body's signals, and tailor your breathwork practice to meet your specific needs and athletic goals.

Breathwork and Psychotherapy

Breathwork in the Context of Psychotherapy

Breathwork, once a niche practice, has recently stepped into the limelight as a beneficial tool within psychotherapy. This mind-body technique can provide a gateway to emotional processing, anxiety reduction, and enhanced self-awareness—elements of paramount importance in therapeutic contexts. The growing interest stems from the potential of breathwork to aid in managing mental health disorders, fostering personal growth, and bolstering overall well being. The section will delve into these reasons, exploring the therapeutic benefits of breathwork.

Scientific Evidence for Breathwork and Psychotherapy

The incorporation of breathwork into psychotherapy is not without scientific grounding. A burgeoning body of research illustrates the positive impacts of controlled breathing exercises on mental health. These impacts include reductions in anxiety and depression symptoms, enhancements in emotional regulation, and bolstered psychological resilience. Some breathwork techniques even stimulate the parasympathetic nervous system, leading to a relaxation response. This section will delve into these research findings, providing an evidence-based perspective on how breathwork can bolster psychotherapeutic efforts.

Integrating Breathwork Into Psychotherapy

Breathwork can be incorporated into psychotherapy in several ways. Some therapists use breathwork techniques within therapy sessions as tools for managing anxiety, facilitating emotional access, and cultivating mindfulness. In other instances, breathwork is assigned as 'homework,' with clients practicing specific techniques between sessions to augment their therapeutic work. It's essential to note that while breathwork can complement traditional psychotherapy, it should not be a replacement unless under the supervision of a licensed professional.

Safety and Effectiveness

Although breathwork is generally safe, it can occasionally trigger intense emotional experiences or physical discomfort, demanding a careful approach to the practice, especially within therapeutic contexts. Certain health conditions, such as cardiovascular and respiratory disorders, necessitate a consultation with a health professional before embarking on a breathwork practice. To ensure safety and maximize effectiveness, breathwork should ideally be practiced under the guidance of a trained professional, particularly when integrated with psychotherapy.

Integrating Breathwork into Your Overall Wellness Routine

Understanding Holistic Wellness

Holistic wellness represents a comprehensive view of health, accounting for the interconnected nature of our physical, mental, and spiritual well being. This philosophy asserts that alterations in one area can ripple through the others, implying that a true wellness routine must address these interconnected dimensions. From balanced nutrition and adequate sleep to regular exercise, stress management, and mindfulness practices, holistic wellness strives to harmonize these elements to foster overall health. This section will explore holistic wellness principles and highlight the role of breathwork within this integrated health approach.

Breathwork and Diet

The connection between diet and breathwork, while perhaps less evident, is indeed crucial. Certain foods can impact our breath, potentially causing discomfort or shortness of breath, particularly if consumed before a breathwork session. Understanding this connection helps make informed dietary choices that bolster our breathwork practice and overall well being. This section will offer dietary recommendations aimed at enhancing your breathwork experience, such as maintaining hydration and avoiding heavy meals prior to practice.

Breathwork, Sleep, and Stress Management

As a tool in our wellness toolkit, breathwork can significantly improve sleep quality and stress management—two vital components of holistic health. Techniques like the 4-7-8 breathing exercise can prepare the body for sleep, while calming breathwork exercises can help lower stress levels. This part will provide practical tips for leveraging breathwork to enhance sleep and manage stress, explaining how these improvements feed into an overarching holistic wellness routine.

Creating a Customized Breathwork Routine

Building a personalized breathwork routine involves reflecting on your personal goals, needs, and lifestyle. You might incorporate calming breathwork upon waking, maintain breath awareness during daily activities, or practice a specific breathing technique before bedtime. It's essential to remain adaptable and open to modifying your routine based on personal experiences.